Pandemic Heroes and Heroines:

Doctors and Nurses on the Front Line

by
Marguerite Guzmán Bouvard

Pandemic Heroes and Heroines:
Doctors and Nurses on the Front Line

by
Marguerite Guzmán Bouvard

Academica Press
Washington~London

Library of Congress Cataloging-in-Publication Data

Names: Bouvard, Marguerite (author)
Title: Pandemic heroes and heroines : doctors and nurses on the front line
| Bouvard, Marguerite
Description: Washington : Academica Press, 2021. | Includes references.
Identifiers: LCCN 2021944682 | ISBN 9781680538991 (hardcover) |
9781680539004 (paperback) | 9781680539011 (e-book)

PREVIOUS WORK BY
MARGUERITE G. BOUVARD, PH.D

❖ Social Justice at the Grass Roots, *Academica Press.*

❖ Social Justice and the Power of Compassion, *Rowman & Littlefield.*

❖ Mothers of Adult Children, *Lexington Books.*

❖ The Invisible Wounds of War: Coming Home from Iraq and Afghanistan, *Prometheus Books.*

❖ Revolutionizing Motherhood: The Mothers of the Plaza de Mayo, *Rowman & Littlefield.*

❖ Women Reshaping Human Rights: How Extraordinary Activists Are Changing the World, *Rowman & Littlefield.*

❖ The Path Through Grief: A Compassionate Guide, *Prometheus Books.*

ACKNOWLEGEMENTS

With thanks to Dr. David Morrow, Dr. Federico Vallejo, Dr. Ann Bajart, The National Nurses United, Jacques Bouvard, Dr. Mary Rosser, Pierre Bouvard, Michèle Cloonan, Ph.D, and all the physicians and nurses who shared their concerns and their stories.

CONTENTS

THE APOCALYPSE

This is the apocalypse
A daffodil has poked its head up
from the dirt and opened
sunny arms to blue skies
yet I am filled with
dark and anxious dread
as theaters close as travel ends and
grocery stores display their empty shelves
where toilet paper, liquid bleach
and bags of flour stood in upright ranks

My stomach twists and fingers shake
as I prepare to work the battleground
the place I've always loved and felt at home
is now a field of droplets sprayed across a room
or lurking on a handle or a sink to find their way
inside our trusting hands or mouths or eyes
the ones that touch you when you're sick
speak soothing words and seek the answer to your pain.

This is the apocalypse
as spring begins again
and brightly colored flowers
display in my backyard
the neighbors walk their dogs
and march along the quiet streets
I stretch my purple gloves on steady hands
I tie my yellow gown behind my back
my hair inside a blue bouffant
my mouth and nose and eyes are
still and calm inside their waiting shields.
This is the apocalypse.

—Elizabeth Mitchell M.D.

INTRODUCTION

During the Covid-19 pandemic, physicians have responded in novel ways to the stress and trauma of so many deaths. One lifted her arms in prayer while she was working with patients. Others found different ways of dealing with the psychic wounds of so much misery. Yet another, Dr. Elizabeth Mitchell, wrote a beautiful poem that was published in The New York Times along with other poems inspired by the crisis. She is a physician in the emergency room at the Boston Medical Center who had felt comfortable because she was used to treating and healing patients facing tragedies such as the Boston Marathon bombing. However, the spread of the coronavirus filled her with something she had never experienced before: fear and anxiety. It was not only the virus that reached into her deepest feelings, but the absence of testing, and the shortage of the protective gear she so needed. Dr. Jorge Mercado was on the front lines at the time New York City was overcome with a surge of coronavirus patients, and when both diagnoses and treatment were yet to be found. He responded with a multifaceted approach, both philosophical and medical.

Most people don't realize that while under normal circumstances physicians and nurses can experience stress and exhaustion, and the Covid-19 pandemic introduced unprecedented challenges. Many healthcare workers were traumatized by the number of deaths that happened under their watch. In fact because of the high rate of critically ill, patients, the ranks of doctors and nurses are beginning to thin out. By the end of December 2020, as the number of cases and deaths surged, so many frontline workers were suffering from fatigue, anxiety and depression –come became ill themselves, and others committed suicide. Physicians like Dr. Schwarcz were experiencing PTSD (Post-Traumatic Stress Disorder) from working too many hours with an overwhelming number of patients. Some hospitals didn't have enough ventilators, and they kept hearing Code Blue after Code blue of deaths as they were struggling with an excessive number of patients. Medical workers also had to deal with widespread misinformation about mask wearing and social distancing which made their work even more difficult. Some physicians like Dr. Federico Vallejo who were overwhelmed by the number of coronavirus patients in the early days, started a very successful TikTok program to educate people about the virus.

The coronavirus appeared at the beginning of February 2020 when a young person entered the U.S. from a trip to Wuhan, China. Shortly after, there was a breakout that few people became immediately aware about. When Biogen, a Cambridge Biotech company, held a conference in Boston with executives from several countries, conference participants hands with each other and gathered not only during the meetings, but also over meals at their hotels. Unbeknownst to them was that some were infected with the virus and as a result, 300,000 infections spread out around the world including two percent in the U.S.[1]

Then there were casualties among medical workers that people are largely unaware of. For example, during the five months of the virus surge, nurses still didn't have the PPE (Personal Protective Equipment) that they critically need as they are the most vulnerable in the pandemic. They were working with more patients than ever before in an understaffed situation. According to the National Nurses United, the country's largest union of registered nurses which represents 170,000 nurses across the country, 3,300 health care workers have died of the virus as of January 2021. Nurses worked for weeks without wearing protective N95 masks and while reusing PPEs. Seventy- nine percent of these workers had not been tested, and 76 percent felt that their employers were not providing them with a safe environment. This puts them at a greater risk of contacting the virus.[2]

Nurses in hospitals and health care facilities are experiencing increased levels of violence during the pandemic. This is due to a number of factors ranging from inadequate staffing of health care services, to stress, fear, and anger resulting from illness and loss. Representative Joe Courtney, (D-CT) introduced a bill in Congress HR 1195, the Workplace Violence Prevention for Health Care and Social Service Workers Act. It passed the House, but it is still pending approval in the Senate. National Nurses United is holding rallies in support of the proposed legislation. .

In August 2020, Bonnie Castillo, executive director of the National Nurses United called on OSHA-DOL to investigate the hospital giant HCA Healthcare for violation of workplace safety rules. Nurses provide health care around the clock, and this causes them to suffer emotional trauma as well. They face many issues including inadequate wages and hospital understaffing exacerbated by health care workers falling ill or working with a heavier patient load than usual, or retiring early because they were afraid of coming down with the infection. The National Nurses United have staged protests, and supported nurses who have spoken up against their employers. Bonnie Castillo was named as one of *Time Magazine's* 100 most influential persons in the world in 2020.

Also the nurses were angry that most NFL athletes, Major League Soccer and Major League Baseball were entitled to be tested at no cost to them, while about two thirds of the National Nurses United had never been tested, and many of those who were had to pay for them. The nurses see it as a political decision because sporting events are big money makers.[3]

One anesthesiologist, Claire Rezba, started tracking virus -related deaths among health workers, initially just to protect herself but also because her husband was a physician, and she was worried about her family's health. Since there was no official data about the deaths of healthcare workers, she would track those deaths by searching for names in the Internet. She came up with the names of outstanding medical workers, including a world- famous pediatric neurosurgeon from New York City. On April 14, 2020, the Centers for Disease Control and Prevention published its first count of health care workers lost to Covid-19. That list included 27 deaths. By then, Rezba's list revealed many times that number including nurses, physicians, drug treatment counselors, medical assistants, orderlies, emergency room staff, as well as physical therapists and EMTs. Hospitals, public health and government officials remained largely silent. What made that study so meaningful was her refusal to keep the victims of Covid-19 invisible, and her goal to ensure that their memories would not be forgotten.[4]

Medical personnel on the front lines are dealing with grief, anger, frustration and fear. Daily they have to confront not only their own patients' deaths, but also their own mortality, and that of their family members. Many of them have felt a growing sense of powerlessness, as virus cases were soaring and physicians, nurses, assistant physicians, EMT workers were overwhelmed, exhausted, often working shifts of 12 to 18 hours.

So far there have been three surges. The one that began in November 2020, had hospitals dealing with insufficient beds, staff getting infected, which meant a doubling of patient load on those who were still able to work. In one case, workers at a hospital in Wisconsin published an ad in a newspaper asking people to help prevent the spread of the virus because if they didn't change their habits, the hospital would be too full to treat patients-and that would make everyone extremely vulnerable to infection.[5] In California where the surge was especially high, the following month, Governor Newsome secured refrigerated trucks, and 6,000 body bags. By then, two million people were infected. The surge was prolonged after Christmas when so many people traveled despite the danger.

The medical personnel who suffered the most were the emergency room staff, ICU physicians, nurses and EMT workers. They struggled to keep up the spirits of their patients, accompanying them through such a painful journey, with so many ending up dying while other people gathered at beaches, ignoring social distancing. Too many people in this country remain oblivious to what has been happening inside these wards.

Now, our nurses are holding patients hands as they are dying, or holding up cell phones so that their families could say goodbye to their kin. Too many people are unaware of what nurses experience, their long hours, looking into their patients' eyes, seeing their fear, and staying at their bedside while knowing that this is all they can do after all the medications, chest compressions, and other procedures have failed. Many of them go home and cry, emotionally exhausted, unable to forget what happened. Then there are the physicians who have to talk to the people waiting in the emergency rooms to inform them that their family member has died or to call them up on the phone to share the sad news.

Because of the high death toll, morgues have overflowed and refrigerated trucks were at times needed to pick up the many dead bodies. Nurses and other health care workers have found that appalling.

The New York Times has featured photos of nurses and physicians with their comments. They are like voices from a battlefield. An emergency room physician from Houston wrote, "patient after patient, all shift long: fever, cough, weakness, shortness of breath, hypoxia, and multi-focal pneumonia. The sound of that horrible dry cough is forever burned into my memory. At times I still wonder how we will ever get through this whole mess." An emergency room physician in Tennessee reflected, "The first time I placed a patient with Covid-19 into the ICU with life support, I pondered what would become of humanity. Was what I was witnessing in that moment, a glimpse of more to come - a singular event of humanity dying en masse?" [6]

Dealing with the pandemic is like being in a war zone with long hours and the constant presence of death and unpredictability. Added to that is watching people die when the goal of medicine is to restore people's health. Not only physicians and nurses, but also any other person who is working during the pandemic including paramedics, is likely to experience PTSD, just as veterans do when they return from combat. Like veterans, nurses have needed psychiatric assistance after witnessing patients die slowly over a long period of time, and without family members around to lend support. This has been a heartbreaking experience for them. Brian Turner who fought in Iraq wrote books of poetry about his wartime experiences, *Here Bullet and Phantom.* Preston Hood described his Vietnam experience in poetry after returning stateside with a long lasting PTSD; and Dr. Elisabeth Mitchell wrote amazing poems about her experience with the coronavirus. She found that writing helped to reduce the burden of her feelings.

Few people are aware of the high incidence of veterans who have committed suicide because they failed to receive the mental health treatment that they needed after they returned from Iraq or Afghanistan. Physicians are also committing suicide. One heartbreaking story is that of Lorna M. Breen, an emergency room physician at a Manhattan hospital who treated many coronavirus patients. She was known as an ebullient person who loved traveling and sports. But the last time her father spoke to her, she was like a different person, very quiet, not talking much. In fact, she had contracted the virus, and returned to work after recuperating. Although her family came to get her, and bring her back to Charlottesville where they hoped she would recover, she nevertheless committed suicide. She had shared devastating scenes of death around her, describing to her father who was also a physician, how some patients died before they could be taken out of ambulances.[7]

In addition, an extensive survey has revealed that emergency room physicians are often faced with a most unexpected problem: misinformation that their patients acquire on social media such as Facebook and YouTube. As a result they have frequently encountered patients who believed that they did not need to wear masks, and that the severity of the illness was exaggerated. As if that was not worrying enough, some physicians face abuse when they participate in online discussions attempting to correct these lies. Public education "has become a job unto itself," said a spokesman for the American College of Emergency Physicians.[8] Some patients have ingested hydroxychloroquine, an unproven medication, thus physicians not only have to work hard to care for patients with this troubling disease, but they also have to counter widespread misinformation.

Psychologist Dr. Mona Masood, created the Physician Support Line after she saw anguished posts on Facebook groups for doctors, and organized a grass-roots support line for physicians. More than 200 volunteers offered to work with her, and they have responded to more than 2,500 calls. Like our veterans, doctors are focused on surviving, and it's only afterwards that they start confronting their trauma and grief that has been caused by witnessing so many deaths.[9]

Then there is the difference between small rural hospitals, and large urban ones that have more resources to treat patients with the coronavirus. In some remote parts of the U.S., there is only one hospital for hundred of miles, without cardiologists or pulmonologists to treat the coronavirus. The difference between the resources of a hospital in Cameron Country, Texas is revealed in the chapters about physicians in small towns in Texas versus those in New York City, Cleveland, or

Boston. People rarely think about how fortunate they are to have extensive medical facilities in their urban areas.

Among the many issues facing physicians is the ongoing scientific study and medical research needed for the best treatment of the coronavirus. Besides the desire of physicians to help their patients, is the fact that the illness and its treatments are still being studied. Then there are the problems of the physical fatigue of medical workers from working long hours under highly tense conditions. Finally, there is the uncertainty, stress, and grief that are an inherent part of medical work. These feelings do not go away, but stay with them over a long period of time. As for the nurses, they spend long stretches of time with their patients, concerned about their feelings as well as about their own health, so their suffering is magnified.

There is also the problem of childcare for physicians and nurses. Their children are doing online classes instead of attending classes. That means that medical workers need access to childcare that might not be available, although in Massachusetts, some of them have access to special centers for children provided by their hospitals. Some work with telemedicine, others prefer to work part time despite the financial consequences of reduced income, and others just quit at a time when the country's medical facilities are already seriously understaffed. An OBGYN physician wrote about the fact that three quarters of health care providers are women, many with children. In her words, "If schools don't open in the fall, or if some other child care solution isn't devised ... a large share of our hospital workers will be in an untenable situation, ... If female health-care providers are forced to keep juggling tutoring and their jobs, the medical system may not hold. And we need it to hold."[10]

Schools did open in the early months of 2021, but the openings revealed serious racial and economic gaps. One half of white elementary students were learning in-person, while 60 percent of black and Hispanic students, and 68 percent of Asian students were learning remotely. In the relief bill proposed by President Biden, there was $1.2 billion for quality summer learning programs that would include English language learners, and students with disabilities. In late March 2021, the Education

Department announced that states would collaborate to help develop effective learning options in summer.[11]

A number of physicians including former and current members of the Health Advisory Committee warned that the revamping of coronavirus database by the Trump administration was placing a burden on hospitals and compromising data integrity. Former Health Secretary Alex M. Azar had ordered that data reports be sent to a private vendor for inclusion in a central database in the White House instead of to the CDC (Centers for Disease Control and Prevention). Even the very measures designed to protect the public health were being politicized. For example, the CDC yielded to pressure from the Trump administration to keep schools open in the summer of 2020 despite the surge in infections. It also followed the administration's instructions to send data about the virus directly to the White House rather than to CDC, that meant that these statistics were no longer accessible. This decision made it very difficult for hospitals to plan for the availability of beds and the capacity of their ERs and ICUs, as well as for the number of ventilators and the amount of drugs needed. Meanwhile, by October 2020, the number of hospitalized patients rose by 46 percent. With physicians and hospital administrators struggling with keeping track of the number of patients, available beds, and allocation of supplies such as ventilators or drugs, this lack of reliable statistics made their jobs even more difficult.

Current and former members of the Healthcare Infection Control Practices (HIPAC, part of CDC) warned that the new database was placing a large burden on hospitals and would have serious consequences on the integrity of the data. They added that moving from CDC to a private vendor, Teletracking Technologies, hindered the ability of hospitals to make critical care decisions. That company's system had no previous experience in working on this kind of data collection, and had been plagued by errors and inconsistencies from the beginning.[12] The warning letter was signed by doctors, nurses, public health experts, as well as top officials of the Infection Control personnel from hospitals around the country. This caused a deep divide between the CDC and its parent agency, the Department of Health and Human Services.[13] In fact after the 2020 presidential election, the former chief of staff and the deputy chief of staff of the CDC spoke out about the former president's dismissal of science, the diminishing of its influence, the changing of its messaging, and the reduction of its budget.

On March 28, 2021, CNN aired 'Covid War: The Pandemic Doctors Speak Out', with several top doctors in the Trump administration criticizing the government's response to the coronavirus after more than 400,000 people had died in 2020. They pointed out that while it had promised to deliver 100 million doses of vaccines, only a fraction became available. One of these doctors argued that hundreds of thousands of coronavirus deaths could have been prevented, and a number of them stated that the Trump administration was promoting falsehoods. Other physicians responded to the report by explaining that the former officials were just saying what the administration wanted them to say, and were covering their own behaviors.

By the end of April 2021, three out of ten healthcare workers were considering leaving the profession. This was not only due to the trauma and exhaustion that they had experienced, but also because of the chaos, their growing workload, and their extremely long hours. Also, over the recent decades, the country's healthcare system suffered from bureaucratic hurdles, concerns over malpractice lawsuits, and a dearth of resources that the pandemic exacerbated. A physician complained that healthcare is managed by insurance companies, pharmaceutical companies and private equity which means that too many patient decisions are no longer made by doctors.[14] The nurses have complained about this not only to their peers, but also to the hospital administrations where they work.

Doctors and nurses feel they endure betrayal and hypocrisy from the public whose health they were giving their lives to save. In the early months of the pandemic, people were clapping and raising thank you signs outside of the hospitals where they worked. But at the same time, healthcare workers would also notice people going out in crowds and enjoying themselves during lockdowns. And they would see too many people refusing to wear face- masks or to observe social distancing, particularly in some states such as Ohio. About six in ten of nurses and doctors think that most Americans were not taking enough precautions to prevent the spread of Coivd-19, and seven in ten found that the country has done only a poor or fair job handling the pandemic.[15]

Then there is the increasing shortage of doctors and nurses that the country was facing even before the pandemic. That is in part due to the encouragement by both political parties to promote the hiring of nurse practitioners rather than doctors as a way to save money since most hospitals are operated for profit. Then there are companies like Optum that are buying out medical practices and doing the same. The grueling impact of the pandemic over health workers in terms of psychic and emotional wounds led many of them to quit. One million nurses might retire within ten years, and the U.S. could also be short of 130,000 doctors by then.[16]

A significant factor to that shortage is the decision by the Trump administration to end special visas allowing doctors from other countries to practice in the U.S. Few people realize that one third of the physicians in the U.S. as well as a large number of nurses are immigrants at a time when there is a widespread backlash against immigration. That decision will cause health care to become more expensive and less accessible something poor people experience, and will also affect the middle class.

The Pandemic and Racism

When we think about pandemics, we need to reflect on the fate of the minorities who are marginalized in so many ways. Some of the physicians who responded to the pandemic have put in sharp relief that it was deeply intertwined with institutionalized racism. More than 120 physicians at the Columbia hospital in New York City held a protest "120 White Coats for Black Lives Matter" to honor George Floyd and to support antiracism. The protest lasted 8 minutes and 46 seconds, and was posted on Twitter. This was the same amount of time it took a policeman to hold his knee on George Floyds' neck and to kill him. There were many other protests by physicians against racism throughout the country.

For black physicians, the protests are about the health risks that black Americans face. But how many people realize that a black physician would often keep wearing his scrubs when he returns from work in order to avoid being pulled over by a policeman? Black physicians are invisible at the highest levels. In June 2021, the editor of JAMA (Journal of American Medicine) resigned as did his boss over a podcast denying racism. It revealed the way in which historically, discrimination became part of medicine. The five top medical journals including the New England Journal of Medicine do not address this issue, and affects the staffing which are mostly white and male. As a result black and Latino physicians have had difficulty publishing their articles.[17] The resignation of the editors has led to an open discussion of these problems. A few people of color were hired, but we still have to openly discuss, and make significant changes in what is now referred to as structural racism.

The coronavirus is affecting a higher percent of the black population who are living in poor, crowded and underserved places, and as a result are experiencing more health problems and a shorter life span. It is as if we lived in two countries where the black people live with low wages, poor housing, insufficient health care, and cannot afford to eat healthy diets, and thus are already at risk. Black Americans represent 13 percent of the U.S. population, but account for 24 percent of deaths from Covid-19.

The CDC researched the number of deaths among young people under the age of 21 revealing an unsettling racial disparity. Of the children who died, 45 percent were Hispanic, 28 percent were Black and 4 percent were American Indian. Hispanic Americans die when they are in their most productive years, younger than white Americans. Extended families live together in order to be able to pay the rent, and are thus more vulnerable. They also found that this is occurring at a time when there is an intense backlash against immigrants.[18] Then there are the millions of Native Americans many of whom lack electricity or running water, and are suffering at high rates from the virus infection.

People who are the most vulnerable to Covid-19 are workers in meat or poultry plants, and those who work in agriculture. Many of them have gotten infected, but in 2020, their employers refused to allow OSHA (Occupational Safety and Health Administration) inspectors into the plants. However, by March 2021, those workers were getting vaccinated. Before that, there was no distancing, or mask wearing, and the bathrooms were very crowded. Since many agricultural workers are on work visas or are undocumented, they haven't fared much better.

In Amazon's warehouses, people are working long hours with no social distancing, and many have become infected with the coronavirus. There are also people who are considered as essential workers and not subject to lockdowns in nursing homes, retirement homes, who work as domestic cleaners, and caretakers of the elderly. In addition, there are communities where immigrants and undocumented immigrants live in crowded housing and apartment buildings where even the hallways are filled with people. Undocumented workers who become infected are afraid to seek medical care because they fear deportation. Among other essential workers are bus drivers, including one who died as a result of a passenger who kept coughing near him.

The marginalized are the most vulnerable. Prisons cannot provide social distancing and do not provide clean clothes and sanitizers. Thousands of prisoners have died as a result. Some prisons have placed people with the coronavirus in solitary confinement. At least 1,400 prisoners die every day because the sanitary conditions are woefully inadequate.[19] U.S. prisons have a very high number of black and Hispanic inmates including over twenty thousand undocumented immigrants. Those include young children separated from their families and placed in private prisons that do not provide adequate medical care to protect them from catching the virus infection. Many of them have died from the coronavirus. A Los Angeles judge ruled to release undocumented immigrant children who were in prison under terrible conditions, but that order did not apply to their parents.[20]

The homeless are very likely to become ill because they are not able to take the simplest protective measures against the virus such as frequently washing their hands or wearing masks. In Boston, the Pine Street Inn created new shelters where homeless people can keep appropriate distance between each other. Some of these are in unused dormitories of colleges that are locked down. However, the care of the homeless varies greatly from one state to the other.

Given the vulnerability of minorities, of undocumented immigrants, of people who are the highest risk in their places of work, protecting those who are vulnerable has also become a human rights issue. Black and Hispanic children have had disproportionately higher rates of infection, lacking access to testing and health care. Many live in multigenerational households, and have parents who are essential workers. Even testing or vaccinations have not been planned for the African American and Hispanic populations, although some places have become more inclusive. In the U.S., the virus appeared at a time when racism had become a major issue, and those who demonstrated against it and supporting changes were diverse, not only black. Nurses found that while the wide news coverage given to racism somewhat undermined the coverage of the pandemic, it revealed the connection between racism and the coronavirus.

Hazardous air pollutants can make the coronavirus more serious—or even deadlier according to researchers at the New College of Environmental Science and Forestry of the State University. That study found a close correlation between levels of hazardous pollutants, and the per-capita death rate from the coronavirus. It was found in a number of counties in Louisiana, and the Bronx in New York City. These areas are inhabited by minorities, and by people who live in low-income, impoverished areas.[21]

Then there is another deeply upsetting side effect of the pandemic. The fact that former President Trump referred to the coronavirus as the "Kung Flu," and "China's virus" led to a wave of brutal bigotry against Asians. Mistreatment of the Asian population has occurred for many past decades, but in 2020 and 2021, thousands of Asians have experienced physical and verbal assaults, and a number have been killed. Not surprisingly, Asian Americans are afraid to go out. PBS news showed a Chinese university student being spat upon as she walked down the street in 2020.

Differences between the United States and other countries

In July 2020, the world experienced a second wave of the pandemic followed by high surges in October and November, and again after the Christmas holidays. Although Italy, France, Germany and some Asian countries had done well at the beginning, they saw their case numbers rising during the late summer. Other countries including South Korea, Norway, and New Zealand had enacted policies that kept their level of infections low. South Korea started testing right away with walk-in booths all over the country. It then used credit card records, and location data from mobile phones to trace the movements of infected people.

East Asian countries such as Taiwan and Singapore were also faring well until the summer of 2021. Vietnam swiftly routed the virus although it rose as many people entered the country to spend their vacations there. Japan was the country where healthcare officials best understood the disease from the beginning. They determined that the virus is transmitted by aerosols. Japan had the lowest number of cases among large industrialized democracies. In March 2020, rather than locking downs and testing, it warned its citizens to avoid closed spaces, crowded spaces and close-contact settings. The majority of its citizens were avoiding those 3Cs. The government also started a cluster breaking taskforce in early March, which allowed it to make restrictions rather than moving between extremes of lockdowns and re-openings. It also has a universal healthcare, many well equipped hospitals, and well trained contact tracers.[22]

Despite its initial denial of the pandemic, China managed to curb the spread of the virus. In fact people who traveled to China discovered that it had fewer than 100,000 infections for all of 2020 while the U.S. has had more than that on a daily basis since November 2020. [23] Initially China censured the accounts about the coronavirus in Wuhan although Dr. Gao, the head of the Chinese Center for Disease Control and Prevention, and Dr. Robert Redfield, the head of the CDC were working in partnership. Dr. George Gao found that it was a SARS virus, traced it to a wild animal market, and established that it was a human-to-human transmission.[24] Unfortunately, politics restrained both men from speaking out. As the trade war escalated, the Trump administration lost an important part of their partnership, a chance to access valuable intelligence about the virus, and to work with China instead of against it.

When Joe Biden became president, the U.S. reinstated its membership in the World Health Organization (WHO), and in February 2021, 28 members traveled to China for four weeks. It didn't go very well. They were told to quarantine for two weeks, and then found it difficult to discuss the sources of the coronavirus. Their Chinese counterparts told them that the virus did not spread from the Wuhan Institute of Virology, but from a sea- food market that further exacerbated their differences. There is still no universally accepted theory of what caused the pandemic. In late May 2021, 18 leading scientists published a letter in the academic journal *Science*, that "theories of accidental release from a lab and zoonotic spillover remain viable."[25]

By September 2020, the virus spiked up again in Spain, France, Germany, Italy, Greece, Belgium, and parts of Eastern Europe. Spain experienced the highest rate of deaths resulting from one of the most rapid reopening of social gatherings. Also there were many tourists traveling in these countries. MIT found that for each recorded case 12 go unrecorded, and for every two coronavirus deaths counted, a third is misattributed to other causes.

In the Spring of 2021, both India and Brazil experienced a high rate of the coronavirus due to Jair Bolsonaro's and Narenda Modi's poor leadership in Brazil and India respectively. In India, there were insufficient hospital beds, oxygen, and vaccines with many people dying before they could receive health care. There were already 400,000 deaths with 20,000 to 30,0000 people dying weekly, a fragment of the real toll.[26] It exacerbated the number of coronavirus cases in Nepal, Bhutan, Sri Lanka and Bangladesh where Indians would migrate to work. Countries around the world have been trying to help India, but that help is not sufficient—given the magnitude of the outbreak—and grass roots organizations are working around the clock to provide oxygen and other supplies and to help people get medical care. Brazil has had a high number of cases with the dangerous variant P.1 strain that has now spread to Uruguay, Paraguay, Argentina and Peru. This represents a global problem that will impact every country until there is sufficient health care and vaccinations.

In the U.S., there was a significant surge of the virus in late Summer 2020, and early Fall as many states ended their lockdown. Then in November there was another significant rise in cases with two million in the last two weeks of that month which strained hospital resources with insufficient beds and PPEs, and staff members coming down with the coronavirus. For example, in an Ohio hospital, executives had to delay some care, and turn people away. In North Dakota, the governor ruled that health-care workers who were asymptomatic should remain on duty.

Throughout the country, patients were placed in cafeterias or parking garages, and in some places, tents were even set up to treat patients. Also, there were long lines of people waiting to get tested. It was only a matter of time before everyone knew someone who has been infected. On November 27, 2020, the number of people hospitalized rose to 113,090 and by March 2021, 8,000 people or more were dying every day from the coronavirus. The numbers kept rising. By early June 2021, more than 33, 000,000 had been infected and more than half a million had died. According to *The Washington Post*, while the U.S. accounts for only four percent of the world's population, it experienced 20 percent of the world's coronavirus deaths and 31 percent of the world's infection cases.

Lockdowns do cause significant stress leading to increases in domestic violence, and drug abuse, while people living alone suffer from isolation. The younger generation suffers from being out of schools or colleges. That in turn caused an increase in the number of young people being admitted to hospitals for feeling suicidal or having attempted to commit suicide.

Unlike Western European countries, the U.S. lacks social safety nets for the millions of unemployed, including universal health care, widespread availability of affordable housing, and livable wages. A number of people in the U.S. consider such policies as socialism or even communism although the European countries that have adopted them are democratic. The U.S. and England's preferred philosophers have promoted the view that individual freedom and liberty is what matters the most. In his book, *The Social Contract*, Jean-Jacques Rousseau reconciled the freedom of the individual with the authority of the state to fulfill their citizen's needs by depending on their cooperation. We seem to have lost our sense of community, and our obligation to each other during this pandemic when social distancing and mask wearing are demeaned as an infringement of our liberties.

The House and Senate did pass a bill to help the unemployed and small businesses, but that federal assistance expired in the summer of 2021. President Biden proposed a bill in March 2021 that would provide additional cash benefits for the unemployed as well as for their children. A majority of the American people welcomed that bill. It included weekly unemployment benefits, expanded child tax benefit, 7.25 billion for a loan program for the small businesses loan program, including nonprofits, rental assistance, and other support for low-income families intended to lift them out of poverty. The CDC received $7.5 billion to trace, administer and distribute vaccines. Unfortunately the bill was not passed. In the absence of bipartisanship, and with few remaining moderate republican senators such benefits will be difficult to pass even though 60 percent of Americans support such legislation.

When the unemployment insurance was available, millions of unemployed, especially in Tulsa, Oklahoma, waited months for the aid promised by the government. They spent countless hours on their phones or computers, and even stayed lined up in tents with only a limited number received assistance. State unemployment offices depended on antiquated computer software to do their processing, and they had insufficient staff that meant long delays before a person could get a response.[27]

The Coronavirus and climate change

Then there is the connection between the pandemic and climate change. Although the majority of Americans are now aware of climate change, they do not see the connection with the coronavirus. Pandemics have repeatedly occurred in history, but now we are experiencing the hottest years on record and its serious side effects, with our very survival is at stake. *The Lancet Countdown on Climate Change and Health* is an annual report published by *The Lancet* medical journal that is issued annually. One of its articles recommended ending all subsidies for fossil fuels, reducing the use of dangerous fertilizers and pesticides and expanding public transportation. The Atlantic hurricane season in 2020 was the most active that we have ever experienced, including several major Category 3 hurricanes that rapidly gained strength as a result of warming oceans and the atmosphere. The most damaging effect from a hurricane is the flooding that it causes. According to climate scientist Camila Moro of the University of Hawai'i, CO2 is increasing the temperature, which is accelerating the evaporation of water that leads to drought that leads to heat waves and wildfires and these changing weather patterns will lead to insect-borne illnesses.[28] This not only affects our daily lives and agriculture, but also biodiversity with too many species becoming extinct, including birds. California has experienced numerous wildfires and people are required to continually wear masks in those areas, and preferably to remain indoors because the pervasive smoke is harmful to the lungs. Then in late August 2020, a combination of heat, drought, high winds and a barrage of thunderstorms with lightening, caused millions of acres to burn throughout the state, causing people to flee, putting themselves at risk from the coronavirus as the smoke and ashes affected their lungs, especially those with pre-existing conditions.

However, although in many places warmer air holds more moisture, a climate scientist discovered that in the Southwest, there are declines in humidity during the summer where the source of moisture in not the ocean, but in the soil. Soil moisture that is higher in winter and spring is declining that helps desiccate the vegetation. As a result there is little or no moisture to evaporate with evaporation a cooling effect. This exacerbates intense heat.[29]

Colorado and other Southwestern states are experiencing a persistent drought that impacts the farmers with insufficient water supply. Scientists testing the snow pack found that it melted too fast in the midst of pervasive hot and dry weather. Eastern New Mexico, northern Arizona and most of Utah suffer from moderate to extreme drought. There have been many occurrences of extreme heat, such as 120 degree reading in New Orleans, and 117 in Arizona and Texas. Even in the Northeast, temperatures have reached 96 or 100 degrees with evenings warmer than usual. According to the proceedings of the National Academy of

Sciences, the planet could experience in the near future a greater increase in temperature than in the last 6,000 years.

During the third week of July 2020, unusually high temperatures spread over the country when coronavirus cases were surging, making it more difficult to protect people at-risk for infection.[30] Haze from wildfires in Oregon, Washington and Idaho spread across the United States, even reaching to Europe. According to the CDC, wildfire smoke can irritate lungs, cause inflammation, affect the immune system, and increase the possibility of lung infections including the coronavirus.[31]

A report from FEMA (Federal Emergency Management Agency) warned that the raging wildfires in Oregon complicated the response to the coronavirus because the evacuations and recommendations to stay indoors slowed testing in many communities. At the same time, people encouraged to remain indoors were doing so in close contact with others, thus facilitating the spread of the virus. As a result, the rate of positive tests rose to 5.6, the highest after six weeks of declines.[32]

In April 2020, as coronavirus cases multiplied across the country, the Trump appointee who headed of the U.S. Environmental Protection Agency rejected scientists' advice to tighten air pollution standards for particulate matter, or soot. This was despite the fact that scientific researchers in the U.K and Italy have discovered links between high coronavirus mortality rates and high levels of pollution. Also, a study conducted by the State University of New York confirmed the correlation between high coronavirus mortality rates, and particulate pollution from diesel engines, as well as hazardous air pollution from particulate matter. A co-founder of South Bronx United, a community organization, discovered that of the 3,100 counties in the U.S., the Bronx had the highest combination of coronavirus mortality rates and air pollution levels.[33]

Destructive floods are inundating towns and fields from the Dakotas to Maryland. Rising seas along with more frequent and heavier hurricanes are making thousands of miles of U.S. shorelines uninhabitable. This is a bad time for trying to curtail the rise of infections when people gather indoors and live in crowded quarters where the rate of coronavirus can be high. This is also the case in shelters for people who have lost their homes to flooding or wildfires, or have been relocated to evacuation sites during hurricanes.

On the East coast of the United States, especially in population centers like Boston and New York, rising sea levels and increased coastal flooding are likely to force people to move inland to places that are higher, drier and relatively affordable. Many people are moving to Vermont. That has had both good and bad effects for the state. On the one hand, its population is aging, and the state needs more skilled workers. But, by late April 2021, 68 percent of the raw land that was sold was farm or forests and so there is a need for new infrastructure to accommodate the new residents, including wastewater treatment plants.[34]

Unfortunately these changes will not only be persistent but they will become more severe because the rising heat has caused the jet stream to lose part of its strength. The Arctic is an area that is very significant for the global weather because its summer ice that reflected the sun heat is shrinking, causing warmer oceans, and thus more hurricanes, as well as keeping the higher temperatures in place throughout the United States for longer periods of time.

Yet another disturbing event occurred in February 2021. Unprecedented freezing weather reaching down to 50 below zero in some places with heavy snowfalls, spread out across southern areas including Texas, Louisiana, Kentucky and Mississippi, as well as in a vast area of the Midwest. In Texas, it caused not only blackouts, but also difficulty traveling, and economic disruptions. It also closed 2,000 vaccination centers, and resulted in major delays for more than 6 million doses of the vaccine shipments shipped via FedEx and UPS, whose flight schedules were disrupted. Vaccine appointments were rescheduled or cancelled in Texas, Kentucky, Illinois and Alabama where hospitals closed their vaccination centers along with county health departments. The CDC warned of widespread delays in vaccine shipments.[35] Also, because so many homeless people were vulnerable to dying in this harsh weather, counties had to decide how to house them even without safe distancing. Texas especially suffered from the weather crisis when power failures and bursting water pipes forced some hospitals to evacuate patients while new patients kept coming to emergency rooms either for dialysis or for cold-related injuries.

This unprecedented cold wave and snowstorm was due to the fact that the Arctic is warming faster than the rest of the planet, and that rising temperatures are weakening the jet stream which circles the planet. Normally, the cold air at the top of the world, the polar vortex, is kept there by the jet stream. But when it is weakened, the cold air moves down into the Southern regions.

In the early days, humans occupied barely five percent of the planet, a number that has risen to 70 percent. How we have treated our ecosystem has a direct connection to the coronavirus. Few people realize that we have cut down more than 80 percent of the earth's forests. In addition, mining, construction, and large- scale agriculture have cleared away millions of acres of wetland to enlarge the area that we occupy. That has opened us up to pandemics such as SARS and MERS. The invasion of ecosystems has resulted in human contact with many different species, triggering pandemics such as the coronavirus, what scientists refer to by as 'zoonoses'. The latest U.S. National Climate Assessment warns that changing weather patterns make it more like likely that illnesses from insects will rise.

In addition, because of the unpredictable weather patterns, there has been a massive migration of people from rural to urban areas around the world where various pandemics have thrived. People in this country who are affected by heat and drought will also tend to relocate to states and urban areas where they feel safer. In the U.S., the highest cases of the coronavirus occurred in cities rather than in rural areas. Abraham Lustgarten who has been analyzing climate change along with the Rhodium data-analytics group, and wildfire projections modeled by the U.S. Forest Service, has mapped out the most dangerous places to live in the United States. That has revealed a significant shrinking of the areas where people would feel they are able to live safely.[36]

At the same time, there has been an enormous rise in the planet's population. David Quammen has noted in his book, *The Spillover,* that the planet's population rose from one billion in 1800 to 7 billion in 2012.[37] By 2018, that figure had reached 8 billion. This has several implications. One is the loss of biodiversity in animals. Another is that scientists have discovered that the large-scale hunting, trade and consumption of wildlife increases the possibility of cross-species infection. History has recorded a number of infections transmitted from animals to humans and causing pandemics such as Ebola, SARS, HIV, and the Spanish Flu of 1918. But along with globalization, rapid global travel disperse dangerous microbes across the world.[38] Scientists have made clear that there will be more pandemics in the future because of the destruction of our ecosystem.

Scientists are still trying to pinpoint exactly where and how SARS-COV2 (Covid-19) originated. Jeremy Farrar, a former professor of tropical medicine in the U.K., and head of a large medical research charity, speculated that the coronavirus had been in people in South East Asia and Southern China for many years, but created a herd immunity. Scientists around the world discussed how the coronavirus spread from an animal to an unidentified second animal and then to humans. For example, in Denmark, researchers found that minks were carriers, and they tried to eliminate them.

Unfortunately, under the Trump administration, science became politicized and the EPA rolled back a large number of regulations aimed at protecting clean water and curtailing methane emissions. A former influential member of the fossil fuel industry headed the EPA. Several of its key scientists were dismissed. Also, the Global Health Security and BioDefense unit created in 2015 by President Obama's National Security Advisor Susan Rice, who was at the NSC (National Security Council) was disbanded in 2018. It was responsible for the U.S. preparedness and response to the pandemic. Its head, Rear Admiral Timothy Ziemer, abruptly left the administration.

Coronavirus health problems and health care

The symptoms of Covid-19 include fever, coughing, shortness of breath, trouble breathing, chills, fatigue, headache, sore throat, anosmia (the loss of smell), the loss of taste, nausea or diarrhea. Some cases are different, involving severe muscular pain without a fever. Physicians found that some people get a hypercoagulable state, leading to blood clots. In one case, a woman called her physician when she felt extreme pain in her legs, and he told her to drive immediately to the emergency room where she had surgery to remove her legs.[39] In November 2020, scientists discovered that the coronavirus is also a vascular disease of the vast network of arteries, veins and capillaries. A vascular biologist found that it damages the interior of the blood vessel, the single layer of cells, the endothelium, and as a result, blood clots occur, starving tissues of oxygen. Those cells prevent clotting, control blood pressure, regulate oxidative stress that is a chemical imbalance, and fends off pathogens. Yogen Kanthi, a cardiologist discovered that coronavirus causes an unprecedented level of inflammation in the blood stream, and it attacks all the body's organs.[40] Scientists began a study on how the coronavirus affects the brain in the spring of 2021.

Then there are the health problems of people who recover. A professor of psychiatry at Columbia University has written about what survival of Covid-19 really means. Because of the pain that ventilators inflicts on patients 24/7 over long periods, they must be sedated for their comfort, and to stabilize their breathing. They cannot move or eat on their own. As a result, their muscles atrophy, and 90 percent of them develop kidney injury. Also many of them develop cognitive and mental problems, as well as muscular problems from lying still for so long. Some of them have problems breathing, and others feel an overwhelming fatigue. Because they are not welcome in nursing homes or long-term rehabilitation centers due to concerns about infection, some of these patients must remain in hospitals or are sent home requiring a great deal of care. Patients who are in an ICU for extended periods often develop PTSD along with permanent muscular and neurological problems.[41]

When the coronavirus first overwhelmed our hospitals, it was a learning experience for all the medical staff. For example, one patient who was released from the hospital was still having trouble breathing, and was fatigued. She now sees a pulmonologist, a cardiologist, a neurologist, a respiratory therapist, a physical therapist, and a social worker for the toll it has taken on her psyche. It was only many months later that doctors discovered that the coronavirus could affect every single organ. While physicians have many years of experience in long-term management of illnesses such as diabetes, they have not had the expertise with Covid-19. That is more than difficult for patients who are grateful for being heard, but desperately want some answers about their conditions.[42]

Then there are people who had mild cases of the coronavirus and were expected to recover but who later developed disturbing brain injuries. They may have blurred vision, ringing in their ears, or suffer memory loss. There are also people who have paranoia and psychosis. Many suffer from pain, including nerves and muscles, breathing difficulties, high cholesterol and fatigue. There is a special clinic for Covid-related neurological symptoms at the Northwestern Memorial Hospital in Chicago that is evaluating and counseling hundreds of people across the country with similar problems. The evaluation of 100 patients from 21 states found that 85 percent of them experienced four or more neurological issues including brain fog, headaches, tingling, muscle pain and dizziness. Their study also revealed that living with long- term coronavirus can be worse than the initial phase of the infection. A neuro-infection disease expert in New York City revealed that about 75 percent of her patients were living with mood symptoms such as depression or anxiety.[43] These studies indicate that scientists and physicians must be continually learning about the coronavirus.

Many people in our aging population are no longer able to work. If they live alone, they need to be cared for, but in this country, health care for people under 65 years is privatized and insufficiently covered by Medicaid. In the absence of a salary, lack of financial resources could cause these people to become homeless. Families also have to deal with this problem emotionally as well as financially. In a study conducted in Britain about people with lingering coronavirus, it was found that 80 percent of them were unable to work, and over a third saw their finances compromised.[44]

By September 2020, when Bergamo in Italy was calling back its coronavirus survivors, it found that half of them had not fully recovered. It was just one of the studies round the world that is examining the lingering damage of the virus. After treatment on ventilators, some patients were found to have fungus-filled bubbles in their lungs. A physician at a hospital discovered that there is a connection between bacterial or fungal abscesses in their lungs. Such patients live with fear and anxiety.[45]

There are also the problems of people who are experiencing a long-term illness with Covid-19, still suffering from fevers and fatigue, and going to bed worrying about having trouble breathing. These people have problems explaining their issues to their friends, colleagues and family. They often turn to an online support group, Body Politic, where thousands of people find psychological comfort sharing their experiences. A psychiatrist at the University of Maryland School of Medicine found that symptoms of anxiety and depression have increased. People who have suffered from the coronavirus for many months often contemplate suicide. However, they can contact Survivor Corps as well as Body Politic for help. Support and understanding from family, friends and colleagues can be very helpful. But long-haul illnesses entail loss of job, and income that creates tremendous stress.[46]

In December 2020, two variants of the virus appeared with the first one in the U.K., B.1.1.7. It accounted for widespread new infections and was detected in a number of countries including the U.S. The mutation P.1 that was found in Brazil spreads more quickly and is more dangerous. The South African mutation does not respond as well to vaccinations. Initially the mutations only amounted to one percent of the illnesses, but by early April 2021, they had reached 27 percent. In late April, the variants accounted for 58.9 percent of new tests. The mutation from India is also problematic and has been found in the U.K. Scientists studying the new mutations found that they were the consequence of an evolutionary process. The difficulty of dealing with this illness is that it is an ongoing learning experience with millions of people in dire need of medical help.

The reason these modifications were discovered in the U.K. was because the government created a national effort to continually decode the coronavirus genome as it spread throughout the country. The process revealed the tiny but invisible changes in the virus's genetic code that gives scientists glimpses in how the disease is spreading. It is also known as genetic sequencing. It is an important technique that researchers think can help end the pandemic more quickly. The U.K. sequenced 214,000 coronavirus genomes out of 3.7 million, nearly as many as the rest of the world.

In the Fall of 2020, the Office of Advanced Molecular Detection was anxious to organize genomic sequencing as a powerful tool that is critical in order to discover which strain of the virus causes infections. It began with a slow start because of lack of federal leadership and funding, leaving it up to individual states.[47] However, under the new administration, sequencing is happening at a faster pace, but not at a sufficient rate although it is rising, and more variants are being discovered. However, positive test samples are often discarded after a week, so investigators can't have access to them.

Mask wearing has become politicized in the U.S. with many states and counties refusing to mandate them, and there have been many protests against wearing masks. Governors around the country followed the former president's lead in resisting their use, and allowing crowds to gather without wearing them.[48] It was only after the massive surge of November 2020, that most governors mandated mask wearing. During the insurrection at the Capitol in Washington D.C., on January 6, 2021, virtually none of the hundreds of invaders carrying out the insurrection wore masks. While Democratic and Republican members of Congress were hiding in a room close together, the Republicans were not wearing masks, and they turned down the offer of a Congresswoman to pass them out. As a result, four members of Congress caught the coronavirus.

In his first week in office, President Biden created a new policy mandating people to wear masks on federal property. As the number of infections began to decline, a number of states ended their requirement for mask wearing and social distancing, and this created a rise in infection cases. In may, 2021, the current director of the CDC, Rochelle Walensky, made a public statement that people who were fully vaccinated did not need to wear masks, a policy that initially created a lot of confusion. Frontline workers and parents of young children were concerned about its effects on health, and that it was at odds with regulations in some states. Some adults and teenagers were pleased and the reactions were different among, as well as within the states. However

Dr. Fauci made clear that the new advice was just to reassure the vaccinated people that they are safe inside or outdoors, but does not remove the mask mandate for everyone.

With many people vaccinated there has been a decline in the rate of testing that is needed to track the path and the speed of the spread of the virus. The average number of daily tests has dropped by 20 percent since February 2021. Although the number of new cases has declined in the U.S., variants have emerged as lockdown measures are scaled back. Therefore, the U.S. has needed to intensify its testing measures.

The good news is that 100 million doses of the vaccines were manufactured in the 58 days following the inauguration of President Biden. By early April 2021, 108.3 million people in the U.S. had received at least one dose of the vaccine and 66 million had been fully vaccinated.[49] By late May, fifty percent of adults had received their first vaccination. But the country still lacks enough rapid testing facilities to conduct routine testing besides local health departments and medical clinics. A leading epidemiologist for the John Hopkins Coronavirus Resource Center has warned that because the virus is still circulating at pandemic levels, testing is necessary to diagnose and isolate cases as well as screening for asymptomatic infections.[50]

There still remains an insufficient supply of N95 masks and PPEs that health workers need to wear along with goggles. And contact tracing remains an enormous problem given the number of infections. In fact, the experience in a number of states has been a complete failure. Some cities in Florida where coronavirus cases were surging, gave up tracing. In its initial stages, it can be very difficult. For example, in New York City, Mayor Bill DeBlasio created a 3,000-person team for contact tracing but there was insufficient preparation when it got underway. Tracing is going well in some states such as California, but is bogged down in others. Successful tracing can be very difficult when the virus appears in clusters following large gatherings, for example among people who traveled to Los Vegas for gambling.

Massachusetts began cluster tracing and it was effective in curbing the spread of infections. When it was traced in a small Native American town, it was very useful in preventing infections. What is really needed is a countrywide agreement on the methods to contain the spread of the virus. About nine states have developed contact tracing that works well through cell phones and apps.

Under the Trump administration, the CDC had been under pressure to restrict testing of people who had close contact with infected persons but remained asymptomatic. *The New York Times* published emails between the CDC physician Dr. Paul Alexander and Mr. Michael Caputo, the spokesman at the HHS, who went on leave in September 2020. Scientists such as deans of public health at universities, the Infectious Diseases Society of America, and public health organizations, said that they were relieved to see science prevail again under the new administration.[51]

Because of the lack of leadership from the Trump administration, seven governors banded together to form a consortium with the help from the Rockefeller Foundation to enable the manufacturing and purchasing on a large scale of rapid screening tests. As of May 2021, the U.S. was carrying out about 700,000 tests a day, short of the three million that experts have deemed to be necessary. Unfortunately, with the surge in virus cases in late July and again in the last quarter of 2020, the South and the West experienced long delays in testing and supplies. The consortium included three Republicans governors and four Democrats.[52] Governor Hogan served as the organizer in his final days as chair of the National Governors' Association. Because his wife was South Korean, he was able to purchase masks and testing equipment for the state of Maryland from South Korea.

After 9/11, the U.S. came together as a country in mourning. But during this pandemic—just twenty years later—we are more divided than ever before. *The New York Times* publishes photos and life stories of physicians, nurses and other medical staff who have caught the virus from their patients, and memorializes the people who died of Covid-19, including nurses and physicians. But at the same time, there are militias marching in the streets armed with rifles *to defend their freedom*, people complaining about the troubled economy and opposing support for those suffering from the after-effects of lockdowns such as renters, small businesses, dentists, and more. Airlines report an upsurge in unruly passengers refusing to wear masks or to respect social distancing norms. Meanwhile a number of states have lifted the mask-wearing mandate and have re-opened restaurants, bars and most other businesses.

When the vaccine availability was first announced, people rushed to get vaccinated. But there were also people who spoke out against it and refused to be vaccinated. Some stories published on Facebook and unfortunately read by millions claimed that the vaccine could be lethal or that it was used to insert microchips into the recipients' blood stream. Those divisions are not only at a policy level, but reflect different views of reality. Even families are sometimes torn apart by their different views, some saying the coronavirus is not really a problem while others are worried about catching the infection. The division is so deep that often people can no longer speak to each other. These different views of reality have led people to only read news from sources that reinforce their beliefs, rather than getting a broad information perspective and learning about the whole world.

What is at stake now is not only the high number of the infection cases, and the impending dangers of climate change, but also the threat to our very democracy that is under assault from many sides. There is the violence from the extreme right groups, such as the Boogaloo Bois, the Proud Boys, Oath Keepers, Three Percent United, and the Patriots that are all active at the grass roots level. To communicate, they rely on encrypted apps and far right media such as Telegram, Parler, and Gab along with Epoch that operates several sites. These groups were involved in the insurrection at the Capitol on January 6, 2021, and there is an increasing awareness that domestic terrorism poses a serious security threat in our country.

Then there are also the conspiracy theory groups such as QAnon that promote a crusade against Satanists and pedophiles, with two of its members gaining a seat in Congress. Unfortunately, too many Republican members of Congress chose to trivialize the seriousness of the insurrection at the Capitol, and shifted the blame to the far left Antifa group. Another threat that is eroding our democracy is that both parties not only clash over policy and ideology, but also even regard each other as enemies, alien and immoral, rather than as political opponents.

Every four years the National Intelligence Council puts out a report on Global Trends. The latest report assesses the pandemic as the most important global disruption since World War II, with medical and security implications that will last for years. It also points out that countries are turning inward. The U.S. has become nationalistic while France is gravitating to the right, and Marine Le Pen's followers have soared. Denmark, contrary to its liberal traditions, is sending some of its most vulnerable Syrian refugees back to Syria. Our country that used to be bipartisan, and where people could come together regardless of party affiliation is at risk of losing its democracy with its civil liberties. It is also losing its role as a world power because countries are speculating that Joe Biden will not receive another term.

Even Dr. Anthony Fauci, the director of NIAD, (National Institute of Allergy and Infectious Diseases) came under pressure from the Trump administration despite his ability to deal with political differences. As a result, his influence as a spokesperson was diminished even though he has been an advisor to six U.S. Presidents since Ronald Reagan, had made major contributions to HIV/AIDS research, and for almost twenty years, was one of the world's most noted scientist in scientific journals. Dr. Deborah Brix, the White House Coronavirus Coordinator and advisor to former president Trump, was widely known and admired in the scientific community. Yet because she publicly announced a widespread coronavirus surge in the country, her role was diminished. But Dr. Fauci was reinstated to an important role in the Biden administration.

After having reluctantly conceded the reality of the pandemic, the Trump White House began to promote the use of drugs such as hydroxycholoroquine, a malaria and lupus remedy that has been discredited as a coronavirus treatment, and the FDA withdrew its emergency-use authorization. There are two other medications still in use. Dexamethasone is a safe and inexpensive steroid that is widely used, and effective for people who need breathing assistance besides oxygen and ventilators, but can also be used with oxygen. Blood plasma from people who were infected is also used. These drugs are cheap, widely available and have been effective in several countries. They are widely used in British ICUs to treat inflammatory conditions and severe infections.[53]

Some first-rate international research focusing on monoclonal antibodies was reported by a group of Chinese scientists. They found that the isolation of two monoclonal antibodies has the ability to prevent and/or treat coronavirus. It was described in a manuscript in *Nature Cellular and Molecular Immunology*, and appeared in an article by Dr. William Haseltine in the April 2020 issue of *Forbes Magazine*. These antibodies are effective in blocking the binding of the virus preventing its entry, and the spreading between cells. They are among the most successful class of new drugs. Cellular and molecular immunology was also studied in the United States. A similar cocktail of those drugs was used to treat President's Trump's own Covid-19 infection with apparent success.

The former administration left the response to the virus up to the states, or even to regions and counties. In fact, a group of states came together to impose a 14-day quarantine for travelers from Arizona, Texas, Alabama, Florida where cases had soared because people were going to restaurants and bars without wearing masks. The decisions regarding the coronavirus were often made at the county or local level. Brian Kemp, the governor of Georgia, suspended the mask mandate for the city of College Park. A few days later, he sued the city of Atlanta for the same reason. As a result, a judge ordered the parties to mediate the case.[54] A school nurse quit in Georgia because she was concerned about the children getting infected by going back to school, and also citing the lack of preparations for isolating children who were possibly infected in a separate room.

A welcome response to the lack of a national planning were the several large stores like Walmart, Starbucks, CVS, Walgreen, Publix, Target, and McDonalds, that required people to wear masks, and to stay six feet apart in front of their cashiers. It was an important way to remedy to the different responses to the coronavirus throughout the country.

Then there were vacation periods when people did move about within and between states. For example, places like Nantucket, which had relatively few cases, saw them rise when residents from states with high rates of the coronavirus traveled there to spend their vacations. Pandemics know no borders, not only between countries but also within them. Some governors required travelers to quarantine for 14 days, even residents returning from other states. Governor Baker of Massachusetts made quarantining mandatory unless travelers could show proof of a negative Covid-19 test within the prior three days. Otherwise they would be subject to a $500 fine. The state travel form includes details about where the person was traveling. People who were traveling from states with low transmission rates such as Vermont, Maine, New Hampshire and Hawaii did not have to fill out these forms.[55] Yet, there were people returning from Texas, having stayed in a hotel along the way because they missed a flight, and who returned testing positive.

Then there were over six million people who traveled for Thanksgiving in 2020 despite the warnings about the danger of infection that caused another surge in cases and deaths. Many people also traveled for Christmas celebrations and that also resulted in a surge of infections and hospital admissions. Also, because of the high rate of vaccinations, a number of states no longer require mask wearing or social distancing, easing restrictions on indoor dining. Fortunately, the Biden administration reinstated the Global Health Security and BioDefense unit of the National Security Council that is responsible for pandemic preparedness.

By the fourth month of Joe Biden's presidency there were sufficient vaccines for every adult in the country. There are also vaccines for young children between the ages of 12 and 15 that became available in May 2021 and it was expected that children aged 2 to 11 would have access to them by the end of the year.

But skepticism about the vaccine remains a looming issue, especially among Black people, Latinos, Republicans and white Evangelicals. Fortunately, two hundred and seventy-five organizations have agreed to participate in the administration's campaign to encourage as many Americans as possible to get vaccinated, a group referred to as the Covid-19 Community Corps that includes Catholic and Evangelical groups. Administration officials found that messaging from medical professionals and community leaders, rather than from celebrities or the president was more persuasive.[56]

Our original goal in the country was to achieve herd immunity. However, 30 percent of the population is refusing vaccination. The homeless population, migrant workers and impoverished population are not able to receive the help they need. Besides access there is fear, misconceptions and mistrust. People seeing others in their social circle willing to receive a vaccination can be more motivating than the concept of herd immunity. Epidemiologists have noted that a small virus wave in a region with low vaccination rates can spill over into an area where a majority of the population is protected.[57] Then there is travel between countries that began resuming in late spring 2021. This emphasized that everyone in the world needs to be vaccinated, not just Americans.

However, because of the changes in lockdowns, mask wearing, and social distancing, by the end of March 2021, the number of new virus cases rose sharply in nine states. For example, they rose 133 percent in Michigan, and in the Northeast states, they spiked up between 42 and 62 percent.[58] Dr.Rochelle Walensky, spoke out about the 10 percent increase in cases around the country. As a physician who has worked with the virus, she expressed her deep concern about the rise in cases throughout the country.

A new variant of the coronavirus called Delta, first appeared in the U.K. in July 2021. It spread rapidly in 132 countries and became the dominant strain in the U.S. It is more contagious, and caused more severe illness. Also it was found to be transmissible even by fully vaccinated people. Just when we thought we had returned to a new normal, we experienced a new crisis with 85,000 new cases in July 2021, the highest level since February 2020. Deaths rose to 370 a day, although still well below the 1,000 daily averages of August 2020.[59] Unfortunately, the country is still polarized with the unvaccinated becoming ill with Delta. In fact, Florida and Texas with among the lowest rates of vaccination in the country account one third of the cases. In Louisiana, the medical personnel were struggling with a fourth surge and straining to respond, with nurses working extra shifts and facing over 4,300 cases per day. They were seeing 20 and 30-year olds dying instead of older people, mostly because they hadn't been vaccinated. Even Governor Edwards of Mississippi, a Republican, urged residents to get vaccinated and to ignore misinformation.[60] In Arkansas, the percentage of patients was five times higher than the national average. Missouri and some California counties were also battling surges. The governors in Florida, Texas, Tennessee and a number of other conservative governors imposed bans on vaccine passports and halted outreach for vaccinations. Governor DeSantis banned the use of masks in places like schools.

Unfortunately patients with the Delta variant that are seen in the hot spots across the U.S. are also younger and without the usual risk factors like obesity or diabetes or other comorbidities. They are also sicker than previous patients. A Canadian study found that patients with the Delta variant have twice the risk of hospitalization or death.[61] Also, a number of epidemiologists have concluded that new variants are almost certain to appear.

What is hampering our response to the virus is the lack of bipartisanship that would help us to unite as a country. When the results of testing are posted, some say that everything is looking fine while others remain concerned about the high positive tests. Many young people who gather at parties do not believe the facts of the pandemic. Some of them died with the realization of its danger coming too late. In the recent past, people in their twenties, thirties and forties have become infected, especially young African Americans. As colleges and universities began to re-open in the fall of 2020 with more openings planned for 2021, over 120,000 students became infected. This is not counting the people who are infected but remain asymptomatic, which is another cause for concern.

Physicians, nurses, EMT workers, everyone involved in caring for Covid-19 patients are working extra long shifts, giving their time despite the danger of catching the virus, literally putting their lives on the line. Also, even though important discoveries have been made about who is vulnerable to the virus, there are constantly new variations appearing. Young children who have the virus in their airways can pass it on to other people. Young people have become seriously ill with the coronavirus and died.

At the end of February 2021, President Biden asked Americans to mark the 500,000 deaths with a moment of silence at sunset with one lighted candle for each of the 1,000 who died. He also ordered flags on all federal buildings be lowered at half- mast for five days. With so much happening simultaneously, we have not dealt with the grief that is so pervasive. It is not part of our conversations. These deaths are not statistics. There was a wife who was unable to be with her husband as he was dying, but stood outside the hospital, and peered through the window, a baby who lost a single parent, an aunt who lost her niece, families that were devastated. A mother who lived with her unmarried adult daughter couldn't bear to stay in the house after her daughter died, and moved to a new residence.

Funeral services are overwhelmed, and can no longer take place with families and friends attending. We have not addressed the grief that is so widespread, and that will last for years. Dealing with grief involves listening to people who have lost loved ones, and supporting them. We will not get back to a normal life soon, and will live with these memories for a long time. Also feeling misunderstood for such heavy losses adds to the grief. There has been a wonderful response by survivors, a political action group called Covid Survivors for Change. It held virtual meetings with the offices of 16 senators and more than 50 of its group members lobbied for coronavirus relief legislation. Although its members were trained, many of them were not used to public speaking. However, their essential purpose was to change the mind-numbing statistics into the stories of people who have suffered terrible losses that changed their lives.[62]

Our medical workers do not live with certainty. Because we are still in need of scientific research about the virus, they are beacons of hope. What we need to do, and what has happened spontaneously at the local levels, is to celebrate the hard working, physically and emotionally challenged medical personnel that work incredibly long shifts in hospitals. This should be done at the national level because these people are on the frontlines, putting their own lives and their families at risk. Plus many of them are suffering from PTSD, and are exhausted and stressed out. They work with compassion and empathy, too many of them working in overwhelmed hospitals, and feeling physically, emotionally, and morally exhausted.

Finally, it is helpful to remember that two important things happened in a single year: a global pandemic, but also the unprecedented creation of a number of vaccines. Scientific discoveries usually require a much longer period of time. While in the UK and the EU, the AstraZeneca vaccine has become somewhat of an issue because a very small minority of those who were vaccinated developed blood clots. A group of German and Austrian scientists published a paper arguing that clots were caused by a rare and treatable disease among people with a particular genetic system.[63]

In the U.S. former President Trump started Operation Warp Speed, and had it funded to develop vaccines. Now we have both Moderna and Pfizer-BioNTech vaccines that partnered with Germany. Months after their creation, these two vaccines have provided tens of millions of people with shots in 90 countries. Then there is the vaccine developed by Johnson & Johnson that partnered with Merck, and another by Novavax. China produced Sinovac as well as another vaccine made by Sinopharm. In May 2021, the WHO (World Health Organization) gave it emergency approval. Just as importantly, it is allowed it to be included in Covax that provides free vaccines for poor countries. Sputnik V developed in Russia and India's Covaxin was being used around the world before its horrific outbreak of the coronavirus. Then researchers are developing a new vaccine NDV-HXPS that is much easier to create than the current ones. If proved effective, it could produced in more than a billion doses a year, and poor countries could either produce it by themselves or acquire it a low cost from neighbors.[64]

In the U.S., scientists are now working to create vaccines for protection against variants. Some scientists are suggesting that people will need a booster shot every year like we do for the flu vaccine. Booster shots will help after vaccinations.

In May 2021, a third RNA vaccine, Curevac, was developed in Germany. Unlike Moderna and Pfizer, it doesn't need to be frozen, but stays stable in a refrigerator, meaning that it could be used in the poorest countries. At the same time Sotrovimab was developed and approved by the FDA. In laboratory tests it neutralized six highly transmissible variants from Britain, India and Brazil. Brazilian, Mexican, Thai and Vietnamese researchers are starting trials for a shot that could be mass-produced in chicken eggs.[65] These developments have given us a source of hope, although we should still continue observing the basic prevention protocols such as wearing masks indoors, observing social distancing, washing our hands, and especially coming together as a country.

By the end of 2021, the supply of vaccines will be more than sufficient. The three Cs Japan created are easy to follow, and will keep us safe. Rapid vaccination globally will be the way out of the pandemic. A number of countries including China are planning to share their vaccines with poor countries that are desperately in need of help. However, this is not happening at a significant pace with even China declaring that it needs to vaccinate its own citizens first. In the spring of 2021, India was caught in the grip of a dramatic surge of cases, and it asked for a significant amount of aid. Some scientists are projecting that it won't be until 2024 that there will be enough.

Until every country gains access to the vaccines, and receives help in manufacturing them, none of us will be safe. Countries are now sending vaccines abroad to poorer countries, but in numbers that won't be able to make a significant difference. While many countries would like to be able to produce vaccines it would take many months before a company could have a site ready to manufacture them; machines have to be shipped and installed, plus the raw materials need to be procured. Then people need to be hired and trained. Public Citizen, a consumer-advocacy group wants the Biomedical Advanced Research and Development Authority, part of our Department of Health and Human Services which comes up with solutions to health emergencies to scale up vaccine production for those countries most in need. The money would be spent on supporting production, technology and the construction of new facilities around the world. This would help end the pandemic.[66]

DOCTORS

DR. ELIZABETH MITCHELL

Dr. Elizabeth Mitchell is an unusual physician who is multitalented as a poetry writer and songwriter. That helped her through, an agonizing situation when the coronavirus infected so many critically ill people in Massachusetts in March 2020. Previously as an emergency physician she had cared for many patients who were seriously injured, and dying from the attack during the Boston Marathon. Although it was a terrible time seeing and caring for all those people so critically wounded, the difference was that it happened and was over. She found that "both were surreal and out of the norm, but with Covid-19 it seemed never ending and there was a period of time when it seemed like that was all we would see in the ER."

At a time when our country is so politically divided, with different views on the pandemic, and states responding in very different ways, Dr. Mitchell felt that Massachusetts was one of the most prepared states. The excellent response was in part learning from what happened in New York. Many hospitals around the country were not adequately prepared. But in Boston hospitals worked together to combat the possibilities of widespread infection in the population.

In the hospital where she worked there were plans for surges, and how to respond to them. For example, they had ancillary ICUs planned that could be activated quickly. Boston EMS would call emergency physicians on the radio, and tell them when any patient was coming in who needed isolation. In addition they would know ahead of time whether they were in severe respiratory distress so the ICUs were ready for patients, and could get them there quickly. They had an ICU team that would come down to the emergency department, something that never happened before. They reviewed all the patients that were potential ICU patients, helping with rapid and appropriate disposition, optimizing ICU utilization. The hospital also put together an extended palliative care team. This team would come to the Emergency Department, and help with patients who were seriously ill and in danger of dying. They helped coordinate conversations with family members. They were an invaluable team for everyone, particularly families who were kept out of the hospital, and couldn't see their loved ones. This was such a difficult and lonely situation for the patients, and their loved ones. People really worked together in numerous ways within the hospital. Another example is the housekeeping crew who worked tirelessly to be sure that our rooms were cleaned rigorously, and efficiently between patients.

There was one weekend when the Boston Medical Center had so many Covid-19 patients they ran out of ICU beds, so MGH (Massachusetts General Hospital) took nine patients that night. The hospitals collaborated, and thus gave a high-level response in such a demanding situation. When the virus unexpectedly surged to that level in other states, with such limited room in the Emergency Room and ICU, patients remained in ambulances until they were taken miles away to another hospital.

Dr. Mitchell also found it helpful to work with other people rather than facing such a dire situation alone. The administration did a superb job of keeping people informed with weekly updates from the chief medical officers about was happening in the hospital. This experience exemplified what a difference it made when everyone was working together. There was such a feeling of camaraderie that made the Boston Medical Center very special. It is very community oriented, and people really care about each other beyond just working relationships. For her, it was similar to the way things evolved during the Boston Marathon bombing. In the beginning she saw patients in the field, rode her bicycle back to the Boston Medical Center, worked there the rest of the afternoon, and the evening. Everybody came down to help out from the entire hospital, a memory that will always stay with her.

Unfortunately each state had its own response to the need for physical distancing, contact tracing, wearing masks and remaining in lockdown. Again this is about predictability as well as information from higher up. For example, there were unexpected surges in summer throughout the country, but Massachusetts was prepared. Fortunately the hospitals still had the equipment they needed by the summer of 2020. They may have run out of certain brands of PPEs (Personal Protective Equipment) and N95s, but they always had replacement equipment even if was different. They occasionally received gowns that were made by the Ford Motor companies out of airbag material. They were strange, but Dr. Mitchell who has a wonderful sense of humor found them hilarious because she thought they looked like shower curtains.

She recalled that there were times when they were out of certain medicines that were used to keep patients who were intubated sedated. There was always a matter of finding a different fix, and were on top of the situation. She was never without what she needed, and found that people were very creative. In the beginning she tried to get a face shield, but they were very difficult to find. Fortunately there is an organization that she belongs to in her neighborhood where she put out a request for face shields, and received many responses for just what she needed. She found that in general people helped each other there like going grocery shopping for people who were afraid to go out.

Unfortunately, as the virus surged in different parts of the country there were insufficient supplies of protective equipment, and the hospitals were struggling to keep up with the cases of the coronavirus.

March was a very challenging period for Dr. Mitchell. She experienced a lot of anxiety and found it difficult to sleep. She was constantly stressed, concerned that she was going to get sick, anxious that she was so much at risk. She is 63, in a high risk group. Plus there were so many unknowns. For example, She was afraid to touch anything and get contaminated. She had a couple of close calls, one where she had a patient who came in that she thought had nothing to do with the coronavirus. At the time they were not using masks, and she took care of him without PPE. The following day she found out that he was intubated in MGH with Covid-19. What was difficult was that initially patients came in with symptoms that were not related to Covid-19, but actually tested positive. For example, people came in after a car accident. Then they had x rays that showed they might have the virus, and ended up testing positive. When things were bad in the beginning, every patient had to be treated like a potentially coronavirus patient.

In addition she found that when you are tired your mind plays tricks on you so if her legs were sore, or if she had a cough or a little sore throat she thought that she was coming down with the virus. Actually she felt paranoid for a while, but months later is more relaxed about it. She even got used to wearing PPEs which initially felt completely alien. She now has to wear an N95 and a surgical mask all the time that is extremely uncomfortable, but she has gotten used to it.

Medicine and The Arts

Dr. Mitchell didn't feel like she needed psychological support, but admitted to crying many times. They have lots of ways of dealing with shock and stress in the hospitals including people who were available for nurses and physicians to talk about their feelings. However she is convinced that her writing is what helps her so much. She could write about things that were upsetting her. She found that there is something about writing that objectifies her stress, clarifies it, and puts it out in the world making those feelings it less of a burden. Sometimes she writes when she returns from her shift. She did try to write a few words everyday. One of the things that helped her was the online "Isolation Journal" founded by a writer, https://www. suleikajaouad.com," who prompted the group every hundred days from the beginning of the coronavirus. There were lots of different exercises such as drawing, music, and writing. The "Isolation Journal" even had guests, including musicians and painters. It was satisfying to be able to read what she sent every day because it was like a creative affirmation. Also she was not alone in dealing with the coronavirus because she talks to people with whom she works.

Actually, she didn't feel that she was alone enough, and actually envied people who were. She felt that she needed to think and process her experiences by herself. She is always with her colleagues and her patients, and comes home to her husband and son, so she needs more time to herself. Because she is a writer, has a left and right brain, she needs the space and time for creativity. There are many writers' retreats throughout our country like the Virginia Center for the Creative Arts that provide a place for each writer or artist to work by themselves all day, and even throughout the night if that is what they need. However Dr. Mitchell loves her job and manages to intertwine poetry, music and her work.

With her coworkers she shared the experience of working with covid-19 patients, but doesn't talk about it at home. Most of the time it is not something that a medical person can share because the language, and the theater in which she works has its own vocabulary and understanding. Soldiers working 24/7 and watching someone's brains spill out is an example. The poet Brian Turner a solder wrote poetry about being in the Iraq war, has two books published, Here Bullet and The Phantom that have fortunately been widely read, raising our awareness of death and dying.

Dr. Mitchell does talk to her fellow doctors because it is challenging to work in the Emergency Room. They share their feelings about how hard it was, what the issues were that made it so painful, and their hopes about when it was all going to end. But they were convinced that there would be another surge in Massachusetts, because the country did not do a good job in responding to the crisis. Also they were concerned about the lack of preparedness n the rest of country

The Boston Medical Center is a very special place. Anyone is eligible to come to the Emergency Room without health insurance because they are not allowed to turn away people who need that care. In that hospital everyone without insurance gets attention and when people sign in, they are assisted by the financial service in order to have a health insurance plan. It is a non-profit academic medical center, the largest safety net- hospital and trauma care in New England that cares for patients with Medicaid, the elderly, or who live with a very low income. A large number of them don't speak English and there are 24 hours of translation services available. It has a large group of physicians and nurses who are proud to work there, and the Medical Center is known for its empathy and for its emphasis on diversity.

Dr. Mitchell wrote the poem, The Apocalypse, after the coronavirus had just started in Massachusetts, and had worked many shifts. It embodied the feeling that the world was turned upside down, and that everything had changed. Suddenly you are looking at things differently and your reality has altered, "a sudden personal experience of your own world changes significantly as if someone very close to you dies, plus facing the impermanence of life, and our existential angst about it." She actually had majored in philosophy as a university student, and has thought a lot about those issues.

Once she was out for a walk and it was a beautiful day. She saw that spring was coming with the daffodils blooming, and it was such a disorienting feeling with the constancy of changing seasons compared to everything that was happening. Suddenly her work environment that she had been comfortable with for so many years had become alien, and uncomfortable. She saw two worlds out of synch, her neighborhood and the daffodils were so familiar, and then the shock of the pandemic. In fact she finds that there are so many things that are so difficult to live with such as climate change. That helped her write the phenomenal poem.

When she started as an ER doctor, her interest in the arts was so separate from the world of medicine that she couldn't connect the two professionally. Over time the field of medical humanities and narrative medicine has really taken hold. Studying to become a doctor is learning what causes a health problem, how you find illnesses based on systems. Professors and physicians never talk about the patient and their story, how what is happening in their lives may actually affect their illness. She has found that this is the whole point of narrative medicine, to connect the illness with the personal story of the patient. In fact, one of the physicians includes poems in his chart. Previously doctors would write 75-year old Hispanic woman. But now he writes a story about this particular woman, and adds what is missing in medicine, what they bring with them when they are sick.

Doctors are not taught that extra and important method. It helps them to be more skilled because she feels that they look at the person as more than just a disease. Also it teaches them that if you think a lot about poetry, physicians become better listeners. They are also cognizant of the nuances of words and emotions. Expressing their feelings improves their work. Dr. Mitchell is now dealing with her emotions in a place where they are not a burden, instead of carrying them when she is seeing her patients. The field of medicine that includes the arts has become a much more prominent idea. Late in her career she is much happier because she can combine those fields that are so important to her. Previously it would not have been accepted in the medical field, but now that is no longer true.

Dr. Mitchell understands that we are learning throughout our lives, and that the combination of the arts and medicine has increased her understanding. Medical schools actually give teaching sessions where someone reads a poem, and then talks about it. Students are taught how to give the bad news that happens so often in an emergency rooms. For example physicians now talk about death. When Dr. Mitchell was in medical school and a resident, students were taught to hide their emotions, to be objective and not let the patient know how you feel. Doctors are now starting to think that maybe that is not the right way, that patients would feel better off if they knew that a doctor feels terrible. Not everyone seems like a cold-hearted person who doesn't want to share their personal information. If a physician is caring about someone who dies, they do not have to appear stoic. Dr Mitchell has found that if you don't release that burden, it will weigh you down. In fact, JAMA (Journal of American Medical Association) now has space for poetry and stories. There is another kind of intelligence, emotional intelligence that some people who are highly educated may not have.

Dr. Mitchell's use of her artistic talents was not only helpful in facing her emotions, but is an example of how being multi-talented can make such a big difference in our lives. William Carlos Williams was a renowned poet and physician. Rafael Campo practices internal medicine at Harvard Medical School and at the Beth Israel Medical Deaconess Medical Center in Boston, but also has written books of poetry and prose. He is also the director of Writing Programs of the Arts and Humanities at Harvard. What makes him so remarkable is that he uses poetry as healing, suggests that his patients read poetry and even gives them poetry workshops. What the arts do for patients is to give them an identity as a person, not as a statistic.

Dr. JORGE MERCADO

Uncertainty With A New and Challenging Disease

Dr. Jorge Mercado is a pulmonologist, and works as an intensive critical care specialist in the ICU of New York City Hospital. He is a most unusual physician in so many ways such as keeping in touch with other doctors in the U.S., China, and Italy in the beginning of the outbreak of Covid-19. He also has a broader approach to medicine because of his interest in philosophy and literature as well as studying medicine in Argentina that used a different approach. But when the pandemic arrived that upended the world, rather than being upset, he found that he was exactly where he needed to be.

Although there were cases in January and February 2020, there was very little information that was shared by the federal government. New York was the first state to have so many cases of the coronavirus. That was in a challenging time of uncertainty with so many people coming into the ICU with breathing difficulties, and coronavirus symptoms that were new and hard to diagnose. These cases posed so many questions as well as needing immediate, and new responses.

At the beginning Dr. Mercado found it was very difficult because they didn't have protective gear that they needed such as PPE's and N95s. Also they didn't know what procedures they would need to treat people with the coronavirus, and to stop its spread, especially with the situation in the first months. In a sense they were at ground zero, because they didn't know what they needed in order to proceed, or how the virus happened, and spread, whether it was airborne or found in secretions. In addition they had no information on situation they were facing, so there was a great deal of confusion.

To deal with these overwhelming issues, Dr. Mercado's team went on conference calls with Chinese doctors, and with physicians in other states, such as Chicago, and Boston. The Chinese physicians had government officials sitting next to them, monitoring their conversations so that they couldn't speak freely about the virus. They were basically telling the team that the virus was seen early, but didn't answer their questions on how it was transmitted, or informing them of what was happening, and how they responded. They were telling them that they were doing endoscopies early, but that it was not really safe. It was a difficult time.

Unfortunately an American expert, Linda Quick, a trainer of Chinese field epidemiologists who was deployed to outbreaks to help track, investigate and contain diseases, was fired by the President Trump. She was the only foreign disease expert that was leading the program, and could have informed the U.S. about the outbreaks. She could have also provided the information to countries around the world during the first weeks of the virus's appearance when the Chinese government forbade the release of information. Linda Quick was removed during a trade dispute with China when she learned that her federally funded post in China would be discontinued.[1] However, Dr. Robert Redfield, the head of CDC at the time, was able to get in touch with his Chinese counterparts.

The virus appeared in China in November 2019, but the physician, Dr. Li Wenliang who spoke out that it was like SARS that occurred in 2003, and was a human to human spread, was placed under surveillance, silenced by the police, and died of the illness on February sixth, 2020. The government warned everyone not to speak of this. Meanwhile, since no one was allowed to speak of this new and dangerous disease, people traveled widely to celebrate Chinese New Year throughout China, and the lockdown only happened on January 23, 2020.[2]

Previously, members of the National Security Council were discussing what was happening in China with two different opinions. One member, Matt Pottinger, was fluent in Chinese, and had a discussion with top physicians there. He then shared the information with President Trump who imposed a travel ban with China in January 31.[3] He also ended the trade deal with China. One of the members of the NSC called ambassador Deborah Brix to return from a conference, and was assigned to Vice President Pence who was in charge of the coronavirus task force at the end of February. After that, the President Trump down played the danger of the virus saying at a meeting with state governors saying that "it would go away in April with the heat."[4]

Dr. Mercado started working with coronavirus patients in March, 2020, and continued to do so for six months. He worked twelve hours, but the team organized themselves to make sure that they had some rest. Seeing hundreds of patients in one day, and working at top speed, he didn't have time to second-guess their needs or even to think about anything else. It was very stressful, knowing that supplies could run out, and that there were a lot of things that could go wrong. When oxygen runs low or cannot go through the airways, the patient experiences kidney failure, liver failure, then brain tissue is affected, and the immune system no longer works.[5] In one of their hospitals at New York University, the oxygen almost ran out. However because the pressure of the oxygen was very close to the tanks, that didn't happen to them, and they were very lucky since the engineers were able to make sure they had sufficient supplies.

The engineers, cleaning service personnel, and everyone in the hospital, were working extra hours. The engineers were building new rooms because they didn't have enough rooms for the coronavirus patients. They had to make additional ICU units from regular rooms. They also had to install the ventilation system for the virus with the pressure they needed in order not to infect other patients.

The physicians developed teams, so that if someone needed to be intubated, they could contact a special team that included Dr Mercado, and the anesthesia department. The stress of working long hours includes dealing with a patient who is not getting enough oxygen when every second is crucial. Also it could be the most dangerous procedure for a physician because he is within a few inches of a patient's face, opening up their airway. He saw significant upper airway swelling, tongue swelling, and lots of secretion. His mask and face covering can get covered in tiny droplets because aerosolized viruses can reach him. Dr. Mercado believes his attitude prepared him for the stress of working quickly to save a person's life, and being vulnerable to infections despite the protective facial and bodily clothing. "It's when events like this happen that philosophy helps you to confront overwhelming situations, and understand that this is part of our jobs and our lives, that we have to take care of the patients."

Philosophy

Dr Mercado has worked with hundreds of coronavirus patients, spent long days in the ICU and was extremely exhausted. Since he is in critical care he was working with the seriously ill, requiring mechanical ventilation, high acuity, and facing high mortality. He found it very difficult. Yet he responded to the death rates with a philosophical view, "in this situation, if death is something that we are doing that is wrong, or that we should be doing, that is one way. It's harder on your mind and soul." However his perception enabled him to work in a time there were an overwhelming number of deaths, and he dealt with hundreds of them

The physicians he worked with didn't have a solution of how to care for the patients who were suffering from a such a new and unknown illness. Instead they focused on the best way to treat these patients. Dr. Mercado continued his search for solutions and programs that would help by focusing on how to deal with this the best way possible, how to find a cure, or a way to help the patients who were suffering so much. It was an overwhelming task because he was used to be working in the outpatient pulmonary office. He had to close the office, and dedicate himself full time to the ICU.

Given the shortage PPEs and Facemasks, he and his wife began an online effort to raise funds so that the hospital would get the right equipment. At first they spent time to find vendors, and try to get a lot of equipment. It wasn't as if the New York City Hospital didn't have the right equipment, but it had to change the ways that they used it. For example, before the coronavirus he put on an N95 mask before entering a patients room, then threw it away. That they had to reuse their masks, something they were not supposed to do, and would have been criticized for that. Now they had to make sure that they created new protocols for this equipment.

Dr. Mercado was intent of buying the equipment they needed. His wife who is a general practitioner, did most of the work finding vendors. They encountered a lot of fake factories that would ask for money first. He has found that in every crisis there are opportunities everywhere, so they were very careful how they worked. As a result of seeing so many scams, they ended up working alongside New York University that has its own vendors, funneled their donations, and received their equipment through them. They were facing many problems, but responded to all of them immediately, which is quite remarkable.

Although Dr. Mercado worked long hours, it was a team effort with all the doctors and nurses stepping up to meet such a huge challenge. He found that without them it would not have been possible. He has friends and colleagues in other parts of the country where it was more difficult. For example, In South Texas, the physicians were contacting their team because they were experiencing so many coronavirus patients after what happened in New York. Fortunately Dr. Mercado's team had information that was available in the New York City Hospital, so that they were able to implement changes and therapies that they were not able to use in the beginning.

Help From Across the Country

Because New York experienced the first breakout, they had less help than the physicians now have in other states. However, New York City Hospital had physicians coming from all over the country to assist them, and their significant aid was really appreciated. Doctors from Texas, Pittsburgh, Washington State, California, and Chicago came to their aid. Ten physicians came to work in the New York City Hospital, and close to thirty in the Brooklyn Hospital. The hospital paid for their plane travel, and provided them with places to live. At that point they put the expense on the back burner.

However, the expense had extremely important results since the physicians could return with the knowledge they acquired by working at the New York City Hospital. Now the problem in places like Texas is more about the capacity of hospitals rather than physicians trained to care for coronavirus patients. They were better prepared as they reached the first surge.

The team of physicians in New York City Hospital also have associations with critical care and pulmonologist physicians, and do a lot of networking. They attend conferences and associations with the American Thoracic Society, and the American College of Chest Physicians that they have close ties with. When there was a scarcity of leadership from the former president, this cooperation was extremely important.

Several times a day, Dr. Mercado had to call a family to tell them that their family member who was in the hospital had died, something that nobody was expecting at that time, and that was heart wrenching. With the coronavirus, a patient could not have any family member or close friend stay with them. Dr. Mercado works in critical care so it wasn't the first time that he had to inform families of a patient's death. But this time it was more challenging because they were not only dealing with cancer patients who had been ill for many years with their families at their side during visiting hours. With the coronavirus he had to talk to family members who had not been allowed to be near the patient, and that makes the conversation much more difficult.

Dr. Mercado has what he calls a more humanistic approach; listening to what the family has to say, making sure that he provides them with reassurance, and telling them everything that that the team accomplished so that they could be sure that everything they could have possibly needed took place. In addition to caring for such seriously ill patients, he had to share the death with a family who was not informed about the coronavirus, and therefore not expecting death, but just news of his progress. That approach required another level of caring, and in Dr Mercado's case, it meant spending time with them when he was overwhelmed with work.

He has high emotional intelligence as well as intellectual understanding, and dealt with family members with so much compassion and insight. He sees himself not only as a physician, but as someone who has an understanding of the human condition, and is able to respond with compassion and empathy. He regards himself as not just a scientist, but also as a philosopher and a person who finds reading literature important since it says so much about human behavior, and life's challenges. He has a wide range of talents that too many ignore, responding to crises such as this one with his heart and soul.

He was always concerned about his family's safety from Covid-19. He and his wife developed a program to stay safe from infection when he returned home. He had only been using scrubs for months instead of regular clothes when he worked with Covid-19 patients, although he had previously been using hospital scrubs. Before entering his house, he would completely undress and then take a shower. Thus there was clearly a line between his work at the hospital, and his house so that he could protect his family from infecting them. Because he was exposed to the virus for six months, he had to be tested several times, and did test negative. Just putting himself at high risk requires a high level of courage and commitment.

The chair, Dr. Sterman of Regular Care, brought Dr. Mercado to the Brooklyn hospital. The chair had worked in a large facility at New York City that he joined five years ago, and contacted the team. Dr. Mercado came four years ago to help transform the old Lutheran Hospital into an academic institution, and ultimately turned the hospital into Long Island University Brooklyn. He was in charge of contacting physicians, and the device chair Dr. Lucia Harvis. She was the one who had ties to the organizations that Dr. Sterman told him about. They were holding daily classes around five thirty in the morning on the status of each hospital, and during those telephone calls they were sharing ideas on how to make improvements as well as dealing with Dr. Mercado's cases.

It is not surprising that Dr. Mercado's life was impacted by a totally changed world of medicine. His whole life had been turned upside down. Dr. Mercado knows that everybody's lives have been deeply affected. When he listens to stories about what the physicians had to experience in these challenging times, he is just happy to be able to do something to make a difference, and to be helpful. He would have hated to be on the sidelines, and was pleased to have been on the frontlines, putting his energy in trying to help people, which is why he got into medicine in the first place, and critical care specifically. He sees it as one of the specialties where you can accomplish a lot by your work and thoughts. This is what he was trained to do, and for him it was very fulfilling. He is always on alert to be able to do what he loves to do. The way that his life was transformed by the coronavirus made him become more helpful to people. He is thus very content that his knowledge and abilities as a physician are so useful.

Dr. Mercado came to U.S. from Argentina in 2003, where he first studied in Philadelphia, and then became a physician at the New York City Hospital. Half of his team quit in this period of time, especially his younger colleagues who have shown an aversion to what was taking place because they couldn't deal with the stress, and with so many deaths. He believes that you really have to separate yourself from the stress, that you have to handle not only your own psychological difficulties, but also your team members' reactions. It was very hard for his younger colleagues. They just couldn't deal with it because it was a physically as well as a psychologically demanding job.

In June 2020, these young doctors decided that it was too much for them and they quit. He doesn't think that some of them are practicing clinical medicine anymore, but understands how this took a toll on many of them. He finds that a person needs to have a certain philosophy to deal with this. If a new physician works for the money or he or she thought that this was the right path for them, this surge of cases took them into "what did I get myself into category." For him it was reassuring, that this is what he was meant to do.

He started training at medical school in Argentina in 1996. In Argentina it is different from the United States because rotations are much more proactive, and thus he started working in clinical practices in the middle of his education in 1999. As a result, he has spent much of his life working with patients, and trying to assist them in the best way possible. He believes that working with patients takes time, the ability to listen to their emotions, as well as relieve their pain, injuries or illnesses. That perspective and practice makes Dr. Mercado a highly unusual and effective physician.

Physicians tend to look at him in his own words, "as if he had two heads." There are the people that recognize that, and it is like a gift, especially, for palliative care physicians. But that is not the omnipresent feeling. Medicine is generally seen by physicians as a scientific practice. Sometimes when he raises his hand to speak he tries too express his philosophical and humanistic perspective, and found that it is not the preferred method. As a result he is always clashing with the prevailing medical paradigm. He doesn't disagree with it, for the scientific way is how we move forward, and medicine has revolutionized the way we treat patients. However he tries to bring in the humanistic side.

He has always loved philosophy and literature, believes that a physician should be reading in those fields as well as in science, and found that such a perspective is not shared. He has been teaching young doctors for most of his career, and some of them can share that approach, but most of them don't. He believes that it has to be instilled at a younger age. By the time they reach residency, the young physicians' opinions have already been formed, and they know what they want to do, thus he finds a lot of resistance to the humanistic side. He considers himself an existentialist. Not a lot of people especially in medicine, know what he is talking about. He tries to share that perception, but it is very rare that somebody understands it. He does not find it frustrating. He believes that you just have to keep on doing what you think is right, and what is the best way to accomplish it.

While being multitalented give a person a range of perspectives that helps him or her see a problem or an issue with more profundity, and with greater understanding, not many people realize why a person doesn't stay just in one field. Often the people that excel in a number of fields are misunderstood.

He now sees patients in his office that have been ill with the coronavirus, and are suffering the aftermath, having developed fibrosis or inflammation of the lungs, and he is trying to treat these illnesses. The team experienced an early blip in September 2020 and they feared that it would be a second wave, but it happened in November. He deals with patients that have muscular and cognitive problems because they do rehabilitation services in the hospital. They have a neurological team that takes care of them, and physicians that take care of kidney injuries. They don't stop seeing patients, but rather continue to care for them. In the beginning they couldn't send any of their recovering patients to a nursing home that is why they had to take care of them. They created a special wing in the hospital for rehabilitation from coronary problems since they saw levels of blood clots in the first months, and thus started with very aggressive cardiac treatment.

Sharing His Knowledge Abroad

Dr. Mercado is not only concerned about patients in the U.S. but also in Latin America where he gave lectures to eighty institutions, logging in from Peru, Uruguay, Columbia and Ecuador. He found a high level of disagreement when he spoke about blood clots and bleeding because he saw a lot of patients with those problems. He found them in young patients, and told his audience that it was complicated for viral infections to have vascular problems, yet very helpful since they discovered that condition in their early treatments. As a result, the hospital system was supporting them by giving them the leeway to try to implement protocols for addressing these problems. But the doctors he addressed did not want to deal with that problem because they were scared of having a lot of patients bleeding. But he found that despite that reaction it was ultimately very helpful.

The webinar where he presented, Lecturing Physicians in Latin America, was sponsored by Society of Intensive Care in Argentina, and another association. One of the biggest complements he received was when he gave an interview on television, when one of the doctors told him that he had a friend who watched one of his lectures, and thus was able to decrease the mortality in his hospital. Dr. Mercado was so pleased to hear that his effort mattered, and that he had completed his goal.

Science and Politics

As many physicians he has spoken with, Dr. Mercado is frustrated by the way HHS (Health and Human Services) and the CDC has been politicized because science is not political. For example in 2020, the CDC removed a comment it had placed on the web about aerosols infecting people with the virus, only to have restored it later on. But he has found that when he is doing an intubation, it aerosolizes the secretions, so a physician needs to do things to protect his face like a mask, and the plastic protector for his face. For physicians, science is about data, and has nothing to do with a person's political views, but just the health of the patients he is caring for.

For him as for so many physicians, Dr. Anthony Fauci has been like a beacon of light because he really always tries to help. Given the many articles, and books, co-written by him, plus his work on HIV, it is clear that he wouldn't be swung one way or the other. What people don't understand is that the CDC not only gives guidance to the U.S. but that the whole world is watching in order to learn what the CDC says and that everyone follows. Dr. Mercado was very concerned that we were losing a losing a lot of face as the top scientific country, a place where people turn to. Scientific researchers on the virus abroad often accused the Trump administration of a failure to take into account scientific advice on the response to the coronavirus. That happens in several countries, but is not supposed to happen here. He has experienced it in Argentina where it is common, so the mistrust of scientists and scientific communities both appalled him, and was a source of concern.

It included the type of medicine used for the coronavirus. While the president urged the use of convalescent blood plasma that provides antibodies from people who have recovered from the disease, it seems to offer little benefit as does Remdesivir, a drug that is meant to respond to other viruses.[6] Dr. Mercado found that they are not helpful. Now he sees physicians using steroids widely such as dexamethasone as doctors in other countries prescribe, and they are inexpensive. It is being used for the very ill, as well as in the outpatient center, and he found that it really helps. He knows that healing requires a lot of organization, problem solving, a lot of discussions, and meetings with so many people, as well as with engineers.

His work has revealed that in order to be a physician who is dedicated to healing, one needs to spend a great deal of time working on finding appropriate procedures and, medicines. He also continually discussed problems and findings with physicians as well as scientific research not just in the U.S. but also throughout the world. Dr. Mercado's goal is prioritizing a patient's health, and finding how to deal with new and what seems like overwhelming illnesses. That he is philosophical means that he is concerned with values in a politically polarized and tumultuous period.

Dr. MARTIN SCHWARCZ

Onslaught

The ICU of the hospital where Dr. Schwarcz works was dealing with a manageable load of coronavirus patients between from April to the first two weeks in May 2020. Ninety percent of these patients came from nursing homes. Then the number of cases went down significantly, and the doctors and nurses thought that they were safe because being on the border of Mexico, they were far from the rest of the country. However in the third week of June a massive surge of cases literally overwhelmed their hospital. Dr. Schwarcz was on call one weekend, and he contacted one of the administrators to tell him they were being overwhelmed in the emergency room. Every patient was extremely sick and gasping for air. The doctors and nurses were putting them on bypass, because they couldn't intubate them given that didn't have enough ICU beds or ventilators. He remembers a doctor from the ER who was overwhelmed, and told him to look at the patient because he needed to go into another room. There were too many patients needing air, and he asked him what he should do, whether he should intubate all these people or not, and Dr. Schwarcz replied, "Let's go there and see what we can do."

He called one of the administrators and told them, "It's here that I have seen the monster in its face." Now it was non-stop, and the patients were put anywhere that they could find in the hospital because they were not prepared for that surge. They had a coronavirus unit that they prepared in April, that they thought would suffice. It was a 20-bed unit that could handle patients in April, but in early July they had almost 200 patients with the coronavirus, and at some point the whole hospital was filled with those patients, and overwhelmed.

They were all working 16 to 18 hours, eight or nine days in a row, taking two days off, trying to recover, and then return for the more of the same. Administrators were also working non-stop, trying to find new places for patients. Sometimes Dr. Schwarcz would return, and there was a new ICU opened in the recovery unit or in the short stay unit. Basically all they had were ventilators from out of town. One night, when he was on call, the director of respiratory called him, saying that they needed to intubate another patient, but they don't have any more of them so they had to put two patients on one ventilator. That same night in early July they had already done a mock preparation for two patients on one ventilator and thus were ready. The only way to liberate those ventilators was if a patient would die. Two patients died that night, which freed up the ventilator for the patient that needed to be intubated. The type of ventilators they had available were not optimal, but older ones that were refurbished. However at least they would keep the patients alive.

Fortunately Texas declared a Strike Force that was organized by the Department of Defense. Military doctors and nurses were sent to assess the situation, but the physicians asked them to stay in order to help them because they were overburdened.

Dr. Schwarcz was facing severe cases of the coronavirus. He was working in one of the poorest areas of the counties, Cameron County, the area of South Texas with a predominantly Hispanic population that has the highest rates of obesity, diabetes and hypertension. The area had become an absolute disaster with an insufficient amount of physicians in the hospitals, dealing with a density of high- risk population. The death rates were very high, and there were three or four deaths in some families. One day he called a woman to tell her that her father was not going to make it through the night. She started to cry, telling him that she just lost her mother and her sister "so please don't let my dad die."

The most extreme case was in early October, when a physician called a family asking them to consider comfort measures for a family member who had a massive stroke from the coronavirus and was close to dying. They responded by asking him to keep her alive because they had already lost eleven family members something that happened frequently. In October 2020, every time they intubated a patient, the norm was death on the ventilator. In another situation, a nurse from the pediatric department called for help, telling him that she couldn't deal with the case of a 16 year- old. Dr. Schwarcz put him on the ECMO (Extra Corporeal Membrane Oxygenation) machine because he would have died. He had so much obesity that he had a body of a 40- year old. Although that machine has a lot of problems, and carries the possibilities of mortality itself, it gives a patient another chance. He commented that sometimes a patient's problems could be improved, and sometimes a patient dies.

Dr. Schwarcz is really proud of what they were able to do in an underserved area keeping people alive for weeks, with eventually getting some of them a lung transplant. For example one of their Emergency Room physician who was infected and was on one of their machines in September 2020, finally received a lung transplant after they transferred him to a hospital in Chicago.

When a patient gets intubated and survives, the travel nurses play the song, "I Am a Tiger," on the hospital speaker system. The nurses from New York had used the tune in their city for the same purpose. They feel so happy when patients get better because they are used to seeing patients die. Surrounded by so much death they need to celebrate when someone heals, a way of bringing light into a very dark time and place like in a war zone. Their recovery lightens the burden of so many deaths.

The hospital sees so many obese patients because the county where they work is the poorest. The lower a person's education and income, the more obese people are. Their patients included elderly people, and people on dialysis. They also had people in their forties who were extremely obese, and would last only a week after they got on the ventilator. Currently one of the hospitals has residents working on a project where they look at the body mass index, age, and how many of the people who die of the coronavirus. Even without any other major co-morbidity, they died because of their obesity. Given that the coronavirus is more inflammatory, it has worse outcomes.

The hospital does have a hot line where physicians can talk to each other. Although working in ICU with critical patients, doctors are used to seeing deaths. But it is very frustrating for them to see so many people dying one after another, and without anything positive. Dr. Schwarcz remarked, "when you are working in ICU, all you do is to try to steal them from the pockets if death and bring them back to life. That is the challenge of our profession. You have patients on life support, and then bring them back to life. That is the nice thing of our job. But in this case we really see that nobody knows." That is a more than difficult place for a profession with scientific knowledge.

The hospital did offer psychiatric help, but everyone slowly started coping, as if they had been climbing a jagged and dangerous mountain, gaining strength to move on. The physicians saw nurses crying because they had the worst part of the job. They took the body bags to trucks equipped with freezers, seeing all those bodies they spent so much time trying to help in so many ways such as talking to them to lift their spirits. That happened as many as five or six times a day and took an emotional toll on them. Not seeing patients improving affected everyone. It was like working in a battlefield.

Dr. Schwarcz spoke a lot with Dr. Mercado with whom he went to medical school, and who experienced the first surge in New York. When he described to him how things were in his county, Dr. Mercado replied that they were worse off than in New York in March or April because they had much more resources than they did in this hospital, including an intubation team to place a chest central line in their patients. By contrast in Dr. Schwarcz's hospital each person was a team who was in charge of everything in the field, seeing the patients vomiting on other patients, the intubations, the chest central line procedures. There were simply not enough doctors.

Both Dr. Schwarcz and Dr. Mercado came with H1-B visas. As a physician that implied that they had to work in underserved areas for three years before they could apply for permanent residency. Dr. Mercado worked in a small town near Pittsburgh while Dr. Schwarcz stayed seven years in Philadelphia before moving to South Texas where he has worked for ten years.

Doctor Robert Rodriguez, a professor of critical care at San Francisco University, has done a lot of research in that field volunteered to come and give a helping hand. He stayed with them for ten days in July, managing the ICU. He was appalled and felt overwhelmed. They didn't want to overwork him, being used to an academic environment where he was able to have some rest so they gave him a ten- bed unit. He would tell them that he didn't understand how they were able to manage such a challenging situation for such a long time. After he left, he was interviewed on several television channels where he declared that those were the most stressful and difficult days of his entire career.

There are major university hospitals in Dr. Schwarcz's region, and he is able to volunteer there and work with them. They have put patients on ECMO, a procedure that drains the blood out of the body into the ECMO machine where it gets oxygenated and is returned to the body. It is only used in extreme conditions on patients that have heart failure, on blood pressure medications, or on patients that are intubated and cannot be oxygenated.

Dr. Schwarcz did have some success stories. One of their emergency room doctors at Cambridge College was working with lung failures for a couple of days, and connected his patients to the ventilator. Unfortunately he himself became ill with the coronavirus, and was intubated for many weeks. Because he still needed to be intubated, Dr. Schwarcz sent him for a double ECMO. He finally received a lung transplant. Without those procedures he would have died from the coronavirus. That they can do that in an underserved area, and help keep people alive for weeks, eventually putting them through a lung transplant gives him a lot of satisfaction.

By the nature of his work he is continually exposed to the virus. He was supposed to wear N100, all day when he was in the Covid-19 unit, although once in a while he would take it off to breathe normally. By October 2020, the amount of Covid-19 patients had gone down. A month before they had eight Covid-19 cases in the ICU. Then it went were down to two in the first week of October 2020, which is a tremendous improvement. He was no longer exposed as he had recently been. Before that he had to use PPEs, masks, and more, which he found very uncomfortable. He was sweating in the plastic suits that he wears in such high heat. When he came back home he would just stay outside in the garden. He was not only enclosed in PPEs, but also ICU is connected to the vents that make so much noise that he felt claustrophobic as if he was in prison.

For the first month, Dr Schwarcz isolated himself in a small separate house. Because he spent so many hours every day exposed to Covid-19 patients, he would test himself and his antibodies until he felt sure that he wasn't infected despite the PPE he was using. After a month his daughter came to hug him as if he had been away for a long time, and then was able to return to his home.

In the summer of 2020, NBC reported that Texas was experiencing a huge surge of Covid-19 cases the Houston area where there were only 1,768 Hospital beds available with 9,765 new infections in a single day. As a result Houston's hospitals' ICUs were filled up, and the emergency room staff members were forced to accept Covid-19 patients. To say that this has impacted the U.S.'s reputation in the world would be an understatement reflected by the fact that the European Unions has forbidden Americans to travel there since the summer of 2020.

Gap Between Rich and Poor

The coronavirus has exacerbated what is already a large gap between the rich and poor, making the impoverished more vulnerable to infection. The Hispanic and black populations live in low-income communities with crowded housing, poor nutrition and insufficient access to healthcare. Many of them work in low-paying jobs and their employers do not provide them with health care benefits such as paid leave when they are ill, or with health insurance. Many of Dr. Schwarcz's patients are obese as a result of inexpensive and unhealthy diets. African Americans and Hispanics have a 50 percent chance of developing diabetes over their lifetime. Our country is saturated with cheap, convenient, readily available high-calorie, and nutritionally poor food whose consumption is encouraged by advertising, poor labeling, subsidies, and the lobbying efforts of powerful corporations. For example, eating pizza, which is high in salt and saturated fat also increases the calories people consume. Healthier food such as fruits and vegetables are more expensive, poorly advertised and not backed by a robust lobbying effort.[1]

According to the Centers for Disease Control and Prevention, "We are looking at a historic decimation of the Hispanic communities in the United States, in the words of Dr. Peter Hotez, an infectious disease physician at the Baylor School of Medicine in Houston. Not only are they dying at much higher rates, but also dying much younger, that means we are losing adults who are workers and parents of school-aged children."[2] Many of the workers were not provided with masks or able to socially distance. That cluster of low paying jobs, poor housing, unhealthy diets, lack of health care, and a good education, reveals a long term and institutionalized racism which requires changes in labor, health, housing and educational policies. For example, there is a hidden policy that banks follow called "red-lining" which prevents black people and Hispanics from getting access to proper mortgages. Unfortunately, this unfair treatment of Hispanic immigrants is only one example that too many people are unaware of. They often think of immigrants as taking away our jobs, which is certainly not the case in an aging society such as ours. Instead immigrants take the low paying jobs, "essential jobs," such as working in nursing homes, agriculture, meat plants and public transportation.

To make matters worse there is also a shortage of doctors to deal with the coronavirus because President Trump issued an executive order on June 22, 2020, barring the entrance of highly skilled workers on H1-B visas. At hospitals where many incoming residents are visa holders, even a delay of a few weeks to their arrival in the U.S. creates a staffing crisis. Doctors and administrators are afraid that the repercussions will last for the rest of the year, and that they will be overworked, and insufficiently prepared should another surge of the virus occurs. As of 2017, there were 2,532 medical residents on H1-B visas, according to the Journal of the American Medical Association. But the continue continued restriction on legal immigration may have made it less appealing for hospitals to sponsor visas.[3] Unfortunately, the impact on hospitals is concentrated in the less-prestigious hospitals that tend to rely on residents from overseas. These restrictions would have prevented outstanding physicians like Dr. Schwarcz to be in Brownsville, Texas in a 200-bed hospital providing so much competence and caring for hundreds of Covid-19 patients in the ER and ICU during their 14 to 16 hour shifts.

All of these historic policies mean that physicians like Dr. Schwarcz, deal with coronavirus patients who are facing centuries of racism, yet give their lives, and long hours of exhausting work to help them. They are an outstanding example of the humanitarianism we so need in these difficult times.

Dr. Schwarcz used a range of different treatments for his patients. When patients cannot breathe, the first step is to use BiPAP that means, bilevel, when he places a special mask on them. The problem with those machines is that they can leak air from the coronavirus aerosol to the ceilings, and can affect the doctors and nurses. As a result they had to put them in negative pressure rooms that are not always available, and if they need to intubate, they put a plastic cover on the patient and continue the BiPAP to prepare for the intubation. To reduce the possibility of air charged with aerosols leaking into other hospital areas, the staff places machines in the patients' rooms to reduce the air pressure. They suck out and filter the air from the inside to the outside and, and thus the pressure inside the room is more negative than the outside.

Patients can develop blood clots in their legs or in their pulmonary arteries, so to prevent that from happening, the doctors give them higher doses of anticoagulants. They use blood thinners, but inflammatory reactions can still occur that are so terrible that they can develop blood clots in the arteries of legs and arms. The doctors have seen limbs without blood flow causing death, so the limbs had to be amputated. They have seen brain damage from blood clots with subsequent damage to the brain tissue. They also have seen clots going into the lungs, resulting in pulmonary embolisms, and blood in the coronary arteries creating heart attacks. They also saw kidney failure from the coronavirus. A lot of their patients who had normal kidneys were put on dialysis.

Now they use the steroid demaxmethasone, as much as possible on patients that have low oxygen levels. They were used in Britain with patients that had low oxygen levels, requiring supplemental oxygen or were on ventilators. Patients responded better if they were given steroids. Extensive studies were done half on people and on mice. They showed those that were put on steroids did improve. Then there were numerous articles on hydroxychloroquine demonstrating that it doesn't work. Unfortunately some doctors and politicians promoted its use. At the beginning people were so desperate they didn't know what to do so that they used it. Eventually doctors agreed that there was no good evidence, and stopped that practice.

The same group that studied the steroids also studied the hydroxychloroquine, and found out that it didn't help the patients. Then somebody thought of giving it to people that were exposed, not in the hospital but in ordinary situations. There was a paper published in the New England Journal of Medicine about a study conducted at the University of Minnesota where among 200 people who were exposed to the coronavirus about 100 people were given hydroxychloroquine and 100 were not. The study found no difference in the number of people who got infected and those who didn't. Dr. Schwarcz remarked that there are always charlatans that try to get money out of each crisis.

In late October 2020 when there were more than 56,000 cases a day, the hospital where Dr. Schwarcz worked was being flooded with new cases and they were desperately looking for doctors in his location because big hospitals were 800 miles from where Dr. Schwarcz works.

Despite the new medical schools that have opened there is still a shortage of doctors. People are unaware that 30 percent of our doctors are immigrants. In Dr. Schwarcz's region of Texas, 90 percent of the doctors came on H1-B visas. If it wasn't for those visas, so many people would not have medical care.

To counter that shortage, the hospitals in the Rio Grande Valley helped each other. For example, Dr. Schwarcz sometimes worked with hospitals in San Antonia. One day when one of the hospitals ran out of ventilators, and another in Brownsville received a shipment, they exchanged the ventilators, sending them back and forth.

PTSD

Physicians like Dr. Schwarcz have PTSD like so many of our veterans do. That means that part of the stress is not living in linear time, but remembering the overwhelming work he did in a challenging period. For example in late autumn he was still emotionally in June and July working around the clock. He saw himself intubating a patient, and putting a central line in the chest of another patient, plus seeing nurses trying to resuscitate another patient that needed to be immediately intubated. He had barely finished intubating the first patient when he had to run to intubate the second one, and then to the next one. Meanwhile there was a nurse screaming that he had to intubate this patient, the third one, and all this was happening at the same time. He remembers telling the nurses to call the ER for that person because he was busy intubating a person, and they replied that they were already intubating in the ER. In the course of fifteen minutes he had to work with three or four patients that were collapsing at the same time, and all of them needed to be intubated with central lines, and chest tubes. Many of these patients were so ill that their lungs were like balloons and collapsed. If a doctor doesn't put a chest tube in a patient quickly enough he or she will die. He makes a hole in their chest, putting in a tube and then connecting it to a chamber that will suction the air around the lung, so the lung can re-expand. Dr. Schwarcz had to come up with a rapid procedure to prevent them from dying. He would have two or three patients that were collapsing at the same time, and at least two who would need to have a chest tube besides needing intubation. He had to put a central line that is a catheter in the base of the neck close to the heart. All those procedures had to be done quickly, especially the first weeks when he was alone without help.

For the first five to six weeks Dr Scharwcz remembers that he had to manage 12 to 14 patients. Eventually people started burning out because they used to work five to seven days in a row, eight to ten hours a day, seeing so many patients. Suddenly he was working seven to nine days in a row with a day off in between. He had to deal with 30 to 40 patients, all of them critically ill, and was doing the most complete work with two or three patients at once, many times a day. Basically he found himself in a situation where he was working like a zombie just trying to keep people alive.

Then there was more testing which meant more people who were infected with the virus. But despite all of this, people were getting tired of staying home, and wanted to go out, colleges were opening, and students were going into a highly contagion environment. There were so many deaths in two months.

Also there were so many young people that suffer from obesity that died so quickly. Diabetes and hypertension are co-morbidities. They had 40 year- old people who died. The pediatricians were seeing the post inflammatory syndrome in children where they have heart problems that usually improve with steroids and infusions of hemoglobin's. But they didn't see that lung disease in the ICU.

Also in late Autumn doctors began to see people who had the virus two or three months ago, coming back with their lungs so destroyed that they had became like fibrous tissues. They were on oxygen, yet couldn't breathe, and they had people that were still dying from the virus that they caught a month or two months before. They had at least 12 critical care patients with the virus in the ICU at the end of October who had just recovered. But after the virus destroyed their bodies, they were left with so many acute health problems, such as difficulty breathing and overwhelming fatigue.

Dr. Schwarcz also sees patients that are left with severe lung disease, but are too old for more assistance or had so many medical problems that they couldn't even be considered for a lung transplant at that point. Even if they used different techniques like mechanical ventilation, and artificial means like ECMO, their lungs were already damaged.

Usually when a doctor works in the ICU and someone dies, his spirits lift because there are ten other people that are doing well and ready to home so he can feel good about his work. When every other patient is dying, five, six, or seven patients every day a doctor doesn't have time to recover. Dr. Schwarcz felt an emotional pain that is hard to recover from after seeing a constant flow of deaths. And then there is the physical toll of working in such a stressful environment without much time off. In South Texas when it was at the peak in July, and August, Dr. Schwarcz felt like a physician working in Syria and Lebanon. It was overwhelming to have such a high number of patients coming in that were so ill. One thing that he heard a lot from doctors and nurses is that the minute they go into one room, a patient is requiring a lot of oxygen.

He remembers a case of a 45-year old man who was a veteran from Iraq. When they were getting ready to intubate him, he said "I can't believe that I didn't die in the war, and I will die from this," because he probably knew how much danger he was in from the coronavirus. He actually had an injury from the war, was familiar with wounds, facing death throughout his time in Iraq. He died four or five days after they intubated him.

Dr. Schwarcz thinks a lot about the first months when he was away from his family. Lacking the intimacy of his family takes a terrible toll on physicians like him. Sometimes they were together outside because he was worried about infecting his family. The doctors and nurses he worked with experienced the same feelings, worrying about infecting their families and missing their presence. For him, coming home was not the same because he felt like a visitor who had to keep his distance. All of the health care workers undressed in the garage, took showers, keeping their clothes outside for a few days until they could be washed in chlorine. The loss of emotional support was very trying when they were facing such severe illnesses and deaths. Dr. Shwarcz feels terrible about being unable to save so many people, and admits to how much pain he experiences to see so many people dying.

Then there was the stress of people acting as if there were no coronavirus problems despite the fact that doctors had gone on television telling people to wear masks, to socially distance themselves, plus telling them about the dangers of infection. They tried to let people know how to protect themselves from such a terrible illness, but Dr. Schwarcz found that people didn't listen. They went out, and did whatever they wanted while the doctors felt stressed out.

He also dealt with families who were angry with doctors because they wouldn't let them see their family members. I addition there were many people calling to express their anger at both the doctors and the nurses. But they didn't have time to talk to them because they were so overwhelmed with the number of patients they were caring for. It's hard to imagine talking to 20 or 30 families, and explaining everything to them when there were not enough hours in the day. Family members were complaining to the telephone operators that they were trying to call the doctors for such a long time, and that they did not know what was happening in the hospital. Ultimately they put some nurses in charge of communication, but that was still not enough given the number of incoming calls . That added to the stress of caring for such ill patients, because the families wanted so many things that were not possible. For example one person who called wanted them to transfer her mother to another hospital that could take better care of her.

In addition, many doctors fear that they will be sued by their patients' families. In New York such suits were disallowed three months when Covid-19 was at its highest level. A doctor Dr. Schwarcz knows personally was reported to the medical board because some families believed that he didn't do enough despite the fact the he had put his life at risk while he was caring for the patients.

Dr. Schwarcz knows two doctors that died, and seven nurses who died in their hospitals, and many who were getting very sick. In addition many local doctors who were his friends were being treated for Covid-19 at the hospital. He treated a number of them himself when they were very ill with the virus.

The doctors felt that they did the best they could and that they had to do it. Most of the ones that he worked with, couldn't sleep at night, and had nightmares. Some of them felt that with just two days off, they couldn't disconnect, or sleep, feeling as exhausted as they did when they were working. The toll it takes on doctors and nurses is invisible and long lasting. Dr. Shwarcz still dreams of someone gasping for air, and chasing him as he is trying to get out. He also has recurrent dreams of feeling useless despite all the hours, days, and weeks of stress in the medical care he completed. Everybody felt so wired, and had so much adrenaline after weeks of working non-stop.

What Dr. Schwarcz found was that doctors and nurses really need to have four or five days off to completely disconnect and be able re-engage with more energy. After five or six weeks, he finally had a week off which helped. He found that the last two weeks of June and all of July were sheer madness. The system was not prepared, nobody was prepared, plus they didn't have the proper equipment, were working with the big unknown, and facing so much death. For first six weeks all of them were alone, but in the first week of August they were relieved with army doctors, as well as other doctors the hospital hired.

Everybody has a feeling that they did all that they could. But Dr. Schwarcz knows that it is not over. When he is looking at the numbers of rising cases in Wisconsin and other states, he expects that there will be a spike in cases in his region as well. Given the way people respond to the rise of Covid-19 is not easy for doctors. For example the local authorities just allowed all the bars in his district to open up to a fifty percent capacity. In fact, people in many states are tired of the restrictions and just ignore them.

Some weeks ago he called a lady whose sister was going to die, and who would be the twelfth family member to die. She had both parents intubated in the ICU, and a daughter who had already died. A situation like this created a lot of problems with the family members because they are so angry. Recently he had a patient who was very sick whose family was calling him, expressing so much anger, telling him that he didn't do enough. He put them on FaceTime, opened the patient's record and showed them the medications that the patient was getting. All the family members were there in a conference call. He told them that he wanted them to google the medications that President Trump received; "He is getting the Remdesivir, did your father get Remdesivir? Now look, he is getting the steroid dexmathasone, now google it, the president, received a medication for acid suppression, google that, and then your Dad got plasma that has antibodies. President Trump got monoclonal antibodies from Regeneron He is getting the best treatment. What else can I tell you?" They learned, but then asked "What else can be done?" And he responded "wait and pray." That calmed everyone down. Dr. Schwarcz believes that their anger was the result of lack of information, and also a lack of education because some people don't believe that this is a serious illness. However, not many people realize that anger is a large part of grief, that our veterans who come stateside frequently explode in anger. They too have seen many deaths of their comrades and their enemies.

They also had some wonderful successes; such as people who have been in the hospital for three months and eventually were discharged like a woman who had been on a ventilator for two months. Dr. Schwarcz had a patient seventy-two days on a ventilator who survived. Afterwards he told him the story about what happened in the Andes in 1972, about the athletes from Uruguay who were flying to Chile, when their plane crashed as they were crossing the mountains. They survived there for days, eating the bodies of the dead to survive. He told the patient that he too was also a survivor of the Andes. A couple of days later the patient returned, telling Dr. Schwarcz that he had read the story and watched the movie, so he was pleased.

Not many doctors spend so much time with their patients, keeping up their spirits while giving them medical care. He not only cured them physically, but also listened to them as they shared their feelings, something that doesn't happen very often when physicians are overwhelmed with such a high number of cases.

DR. EDUARDO MIRELESS

Cleveland Clinic

Dr. Eduardo Mireless works in a hospital complex that has the number two rating as the best in the country, Cleveland Clinic. It runs a 170 acres campus as well as 11 hospitals, 19 family health centers in Northeast Ohio as well as hospitals in Florida and Nevada. People from around the country come to the Cleveland Clinic, and its hospitals have helipads for flights. Cleveland Clinic is also an international organization that operates in Abu Dhabi as well as two clinic locations in Toronto, Canada, and opened one in London, England in 2021. The Clinic is consistently regarded as one of the top hospital systems in the United States, and in the world, and is well known particularly in technological management systems. It is the best hospital for cardiology, and has expertise in a number of important fields.

It also has a Cleveland Clinic Lerner College of Medicine, a five-year medical school program affiliated with the Case Western Reserve School of Medicine with 32 students per class, each receiving a scholarship for full tuition and fees. While traditional medical schools in the U.S. are four-year programs, the extra year in the program is dedicated to a year of research. The curriculum is notable for its lack of class rank, pre-clinical or clinical grading, or end-of-course examinations.

While Dr. Mireless faced three surges in the coronavirus, he was working in a first rate hospital system with adequate supplies, PPEs, and talented co-workers as well as being able to keep abreast of the various demands by partnering with the other hospitals. There are 1200 beds where he works.

The advisor to governor Mike DeWine, Amy Acton, helped prepare for the surge very early by ordering lockdowns, and imposing stay at home orders. She had a lot of support from the medical establishment. But as time passed, people started complaining about the lockdown, wearing masks, and social distancing as in so many other states, and she received threats. As cases of the coronavirus rose in every county in Ohio, Mike DeWine went on the air to tell people to wear masks and socially distance which resulted in a pushback, and people wanting to impeach him. Because of that response, healthcare workers often felt safer in the hospital.

Meanwhile, Dr. Mireless dealt with long hours, and devoted himself to hard work plus a number of challenges. He felt fortunate to be surrounded by so much support and competence. Unfortunately there are many hospitals that are not sufficiently equipped for patients who can no longer survive on intubators and need ECMOs (extracorporeal membrane oxygenation) that allows their lungs to rest while the machines infuses oxygen in their blood. While a number of states created surge lines to co-ordinate patient care, too many of them were not prepared to do so which caused the needless death of numerous patients.

Yet during the third surge Dr. Mireless was straining, and the Cleveland Clinic was trying to preserve enough personnel. The surge affected everything including the number of beds, not at the crisis level, but straining his peers and his team. He was working in the ICU since March 13, 2020. One of the rules in place was how to keep safe when entering a room, and working with a patient who has the coronavirus. However, in the beginning, there was a lot of fear in the community, yet he found that the response was first rate.

Then restaurants began to open as well as many small businesses and retail stores despite the rules. People had lost their fear and were meeting in groups. That created the second surge in July and August of 2020. November and December was very challenging. It required creating a balance between caring for the community, and patients affected by the pandemic.

The physicians were well prepared by working together, and holding meetings every hour to arrange their care that is helpful given that their large staff is active in clinical care. In the ICU where Dr. Mireless works they usually see 5,000 patients a year, and thus dealt with other illnesses that are dangerous. Because of their experience during the initial period of learning about the new virus, they felt more comfortable in their work.

From the beginning they were having trials on the therapies available. As for innovation he also sees difficulties because there have been a lot of opinions about various medications, and lack of evidence for medicines that have hurt patients, such as hydroxycholoroquine, a malaria and lupus drug. Now they give steroids to patients who are very ill, and patients that meet certain criteria receive other medications such as blood plasma from infected people, and stem cells. He and his team believe that they have to have a balance between early and later responses. He found that there is so much misinformation that is circulating, that people have platforms to promote certain responses without the proper evidence.

In the early months of Dr. Mireless's work in the ICU he followed the routine of doctors and nurses throughout the country, living separately from his family, showering and changing when he came home. Yet in December he was exhausted given the number of patients he was seeing that surpassed the previous peaks. He was able to take a few weeks off which was more than helpful.

Despite Cleveland Clinic's resources, its healthcare workers who work 12 hours in a row, experienced fear and uncertainty when it came to their families. Dr. Mireless was also concerned about how it could affect his team, and his community because one of them could have caught the infection. Then there was the issue of childcare because since so many schools were closed, parents had to find a trusted person to fill the gap at a time when so many of them are unable to stay home. He found that women doctors, and nurses suffered from the strain of changes in their routines. There was also the issue of social activities, of getting together with friends and sharing experiences that would help the strains of work among the seriously ill and dying.

He and his wife who is also a doctor, have three children who are nine, 11, and 13 years old. It was very hard for them to live through so many changes in their lives. They went through learning online after their schools closed, and didn't see any of their friends. Then they were able to have hybrid attendance. As of 2021 they were in their public schools full time. In the early phase, he and his wife took them out as much as possible for sports such as skiing or walking in the mountains, anything to get them out of the house.

Their healthcare workers were still experiencing the stress of seeing new patients with severe health problems from the coronavirus, but unable to be with their families at their bedsides or visiting them. To be alone and dealing with such a multifaceted and painful illness is overwhelming.

Dr. Mireless is uncomfortable with the stress their medical caregivers experience, and in his words "as well as dealing with their careers eclipsed by working with the virus, a multilevel and multidimensional effort for the members and directors of the unit, I try to reduce the strain as much as possible by making operations as efficient, and easier for the teams so they don't have to deal with these stresses for working with covid-19 patients."

Caring for Caregivers provides them with support from psychologists creating environments to help them deal with these issues, as well as many hotlines they can call for help. These are anonymous because there is some stigma in dealing with these problems. Doctors are expected to be very strong and generally don't like to have people know that they need help. But the Caring for Caregivers Dr. Mireless explains "are trying to normalize grief and to make resources available for everyone." He sees the expectation of doctors as enormous, and that is it hard for them to admit that they are dealing with grief, anxiety, so many deaths as well as with fear. He has found that such support helps lessen the burnout. When they are dealing with deaths every day, and such a new illness that affects every single organ, plus new medications, psychological support is extremely important.

Plus they were able to have the staff that they needed when respiratory therapists were very much in demand. They had travel nurses arrive to help them, critical care physicians, and skilled nurses for services in the ICU. People that were doing administrative jobs also joined them in the ICU from other areas of the hospital. In the early period, the staff thought it would be like the outbreak in New York City, training so many people. But they had enough for the second and third surge because they had discussed and established how they were going to deal with these demanding situations.

Cleveland Clinic covers Northeast Ohio that also includes 12 hospitals. They helped each other respond to the coronavirus. Also they were flexible enough to reach out to each other when any one of the doctors and nurses were overloaded with patients, unlike places that have only one hospital. However in Massachusetts, at the beginning of the pandemic, hospitals in Boston that were not connected did help each other out with sharing their beds, and physicians, communicating by radio.

Messaging About The Coronavirus

Dr. Mireless is also concerned about the way people receive information about the virus because it can be demoralizing or encouraging. He sees the rhetoric and messaging that comes from the federal government as key, and how the message is aligned. Because the previous administration left the policies for the pandemic up to the states, there is a wide difference not only between them, but also in the counties within them. It meant that it took a great deal of time to get their policies coordinated. For example North and South Dakota did not require the protocols for prevention, and their per capita death rate was 34 percent higher than the national average, and 13 percent of their population had a confirmed case although that declined in the winter of 2020.[1] He also believes that a big part is regional and age based, that dealing with the pandemic is not about freedom as so many people claim in marches, and on Facebook, but about survival.

In fact the House Committee on Energy and Commerce held a hearing on March 20, 2021, that featured an appearance by Facebook CEO Mark Zuckerberg, plus CEOs of Google and Twitter to testify about falsehoods regarding the pandemic, including anti-vaxxers. The algorithms spread hate speech and disinformation about the virus. Meanwhile thousands of local newspapers have closed because of finances with the result that reporters who earned Pulitzer prizes were fired, so the social media is very prominent and open to misinformation. Since we are all connected on the internet, Dr. Mireless sees how the way these messages are conveyed affects our behavior.

What annoys him is seeing videos of people going to the beach and partying. He remembers a very upsetting event, a large wedding that was celebrated in his community that infected people, causing some of them to die. He believes that the most important civic duty we have is to care for each other, and that we need to hear that from the top and from influential people. It does happen in both grass roots' and national organizations, but they are not widely publicized.

Hope

Dr. Mireless sees the vaccinations that are occurring throughout the country as a much needed source of hope. Millions of healthcare workers have received them as well as our adult population, and the administration had sufficient vaccinations for everyone in our country by the end of May. The pharmacy companies worked on a new vaccine for children that was available by the end of May. Pfizer is the only manufacturer whose pediatric vaccine trials have progressed to have data on elementary school-age children younger than 12 by the end of the summer of 2021. It will bring stability to the education system, and parents' work schedules as well as keeping children safe. Moderna is still enrolling participants in its trial for adolescents from 12 to 18 years old. As of early February the CDC tracked more than 2,000 cases of multi-system inflammatory syndrome in children. a serious condition associated with the coronavirus that can create cardiac problems, and kidney injury.[2]

There is a certain percentage of our population that is hesitant about receiving vaccinations as there is in many other countries. In the U.S., 15 percent of our military refuse to take them, and so do some of our health care workers. For example, nurses and long-term care staff such as people who work in nursing homes do not feel well treated because their pay is low, thus refusing vaccines is a way of dealing with their anger. For many other people hesitancy is very complex because people interpret vaccines based on their own experiences, relationships and trust of authority.[3] Some people prefer a spiritual approach. We would need to vaccinate 60 to 70 percent of our population, continue wearing masks, and socially distance to achieve a herd immunity. Dr Mireless also finds that what will stop the spread of the coronavirus are the preventive measures of staying at home, wearing masks, and washing our hands.

Governor DeWine was committed to helping the people in his state and consulted with elected officials and medical and scientific experts. Ohio was also the first state to close schools. Then the state had too many vaccines and wanted to motivate people to get vaccinated. By the end of April, Governor DeWine created Vax-a-Million, a lottery which awards one million to five vaccinated state residents and a full scholarship to one of the state's public colleges to five immunized teenagers. It generated a 28 percent increase in Ohio's vaccination rate.[4]

President Biden's worked very hard to provide enough vaccines. He invoked the Defense Production Act to increase supplies as did President Trump, marshaled federal resources to increase the number of vaccine sites, and shipped them directly to local health centers in underserved communities. He was also trying to deal with the distrust in the Black community that is not surprising given its long history of unethical medical treatment. The DHH (Department of Health and Human Services) promoted ads in 2,300 radio stations, in minority newspapers, and gathered experts to work with the Black Coalition Against Covid-19. The CDC funded campaigns by the National Urban League, the Conference of National Black Churches as well as partnering with retired football stars.[5] In the early months of the rollout of vaccines, there was confusion and difficulty in getting a site, and a time for so many people.

At Dr. Mireless's hospital, they first vaccinated people who had the highest risk of exposure, including the Emergency Department. However everyone was included, not just doctors, nurses, respiratory therapists, but people cleaning the rooms, and administrators. There was more focus on the team. Then they moved through different areas depending on their involvement in taking care of the patients. He is well aware that there was a lack of guidance in other locations, that each organization has different nuances that need to be taken into account, and that each health system has its own priorities.

Dr. Mireless believes that in order to curtail the pandemic we should get everyone in the world vaccinated, and see ourselves as part of a global community. He would like us to lead the way, and is concerned that with the coronavirus, borders are non-existent. The assistant director at Duke Global Innovation Center found that there will not be enough vaccines for global coverage until 2023. The WHO warned of the dangers of wealthier countries prioritizing nationalism. Also while countries have rushed to close their borders, variants are already spreading to dozens of nations. The variants from South Africa and

Brazil appeared in North Carolina, New York, and Massachusetts that didn't have any travelers from those countries. The director of global delivery programs at the Bill and Melinda Gates Foundation pointed out that by the end of 2021, 75 percent of the population in high income countries will be vaccinated compared to 25 percent in poor countries.

Covax, a non-profit group formed by a group of international organizations whose goal is to provide vaccines, has reached out to 190 countries. Unfortunately many of them are making deals with drug companies that could drive up prices and delay delivery from Covax. The response of each country in Africa varies with South Africa promoting the use of masks.[6] Fortunately in the Spring of 2021, Covax signed an agreement with Gavi, the Vaccine Alliance in December, 2020. In 2021 100 million doses were available with the remaining 300 million in 2022.[7]

In February 2021, President Biden spoke about plans to boost international vaccine production, and distribution with leaders of the Group of Seven major economies. But so far the U.S. has been seen as a vaccine nationalist because after vaccinating most of its population it still had millions of excess doses. The U.N. Secretary General told a meeting of the Security Council that not a single dose of the vaccine had been delivered to 130 countries. In response the White House announced that President Biden would pledge an initial two billion to be used through Covax, and then another two billion over the next two years after other donors honor their commitments.[8] Thus the next two billion is not assured. We have to work hard to move beyond our former nationalism, and realize that until everyone is vaccinated, we cannot assure our own health.

The major pharmaceutical companies that have developed vaccines want to keep their trade secrets to preserve their profits, and their incentive for future development. But the poorer countries such as South Africa cannot wait for the shots, and are upset that Western companies have monopolized them by buying existing supplies. As a result they want to have an emergency waiver of intellectual property rights for vaccines and the much needed medical supplies for the coronavirus.[9] In the late 1990s when there was the crisis of HIV/AIDS, the World Trade

Organization created an agreement on trade related aspects of intellectual property rights which the U.S. signed in 2003, and that could be a way of sharing our knowledge of the vaccines. President Biden initially blocked India's and South Africa's request for a temporary waiver to an international intellectual property agreement that would give poorer countries access to generic versions of coronavirus vaccines and treatments.[10] He discussed it at length with Dr. Fauci in a way that ultimately led to our contribution.

It is interesting to note that Israel is sharing its vaccines with a number of other countries as a political advantage, something that is not unusual, and is referred to as soft power where rich countries seek to influence countries that have little access to them. It also promised to send tens of thousands doses to it's enemy Syria in exchange for the return of an Israeli detained there. China, India and Russia have donated thousands of vaccine doses to their neighbors for similar reasons.[11] Also China and Russia have used their soft power through these doses throughout the world. For example after Russia donated to Mexico, President Andrez Manuel Lopez Obrador invited him to visit Mexico when he thanked him over the phone. Then China started a discussion with Paraguay to donate vaccines that were desperately needed, giving it leverage over Taiwan that has helped it in so many ways. Paraguay is one of the few countries that have diplomatic relations with Taiwan as a separate country not part of "one China." In March 2021, President Biden made a diplomatic arrangement with the Mexican president that would share vaccines with Mexico in order to have help with the immigrants at our border, while his aides were denying that it was an arrangement. He also shared vaccines with Canada. But supporting Covax is a moral and much needed decision that will keep not only our country, but the whole world safe because they are dependent on each other.

At that time our country partnered with India, Japan and Australia to expand global vaccine manufacturing, including financial support for a major vaccine manufacturer in India to produce a billion doses by 2022. It is called the Quad Vaccine Partnership with each country involving different commitments. They also formed a Quad Vaccine Experts Group of scientists and government officials addressing manufacturing efforts and financing.

However, in the Spring of 2021, India, a country with a high level of vaccines was overwhelmed with cases with almost half of the highest global rate of coronavirus. Ironically less than two percent of the population was fully vaccinated and less than 10 percent received one dose.[12] Nor were the hospitals prepared, struggling with insufficient oxygen and hospital beds while people were dying as they waited to be admitted. Cremation ceremonies were jammed and happening around the country. Countries around the world responded. President Biden sent two military transport planes to India with oxygen cylinders, rapid diagnostic tests, vaccine materials, drugs, ventilators and PPEs. In early May after much discussion, and disagreement with the pharmacy companies, he decided to share the formula for making vaccines with India. The German government airlifted three mobile oxygen generation plants. Pakistan, Russia and China also provided help.[13]

Although we have more vaccines than we need, President. Biden initially rejected a demand from liberal democrats to give away excess doses, but promised to send some of them to India. Meanwhile our government was dealing with the reluctance of large sectors of the population to take them. There may be obstacles, but there are also successes that we could rely on to assure global health.

Regardless of all of the problems our country is facing with the coronavirus, climate change, and the economy, Dr. Mireless is a committed physician. He feels that despite everything, he learned a lot about himself, his community and the world. In spite of feeling guilty of being in such an excellent situation that is so different from many other settings, he feels fortunate to work with a group of people who have responded in such a responsible way, He is hopeful about the future because of what he refers to as *this island of behavior,* and he is certain that it is not only the Cleveland Clinic that will steer us through the pandemic.

DR. FEDERICO VALLEJO

Dr. Federico Vallejo works at the South Texas Health System that includes the MacAllen Medical Hospital, the Heart Hospital, and the Edinburgh Regional Hospital. He is a pulmonologist, critical care and internal medicine physician as well as a sleep specialist, and works in the ICU. He is part of a group of doctors that spends one week at the hospital, and one week in their offices. When the pandemic arrived there was a tsunami of patients, and they had to close their offices. He was used to attending to 15 or 17 patients, but suddenly they were seeing 70 or 80 patients every day. He was working from eight o'clock in the morning to very late at night, and some days from seven a.m. to nine p.m. It was very demanding because often they would receive calls at night for more help. On the weekends they had four doctors on call, which meant that they were working every other weekend. It was physically and mentally exhausting.

In the beginning, March, April, May, June and July 2020, when they were overwhelmed with patients, they didn't have help from other hospitals. Also they didn't know much about the coronavirus, and had to learn how to operate as health care workers. During the worst part of the pandemic the hospital was filled with eighty percent of coronavirus patients. As so many physicians Dr. Vallejo didn't want to infect his family, and thus was living alone connecting with them by FaceTime or over the phone. Despite his long hours at the hospital he missed his wife and three children so much.

He used that time to read constantly about the pandemic because there was so much information coming in. He was also calling other doctors throughout the country so that they could collaborate and contacted the most prominent institutions such as the Brigham and Women's Hospital in Boston, his peers at the University of Massachusetts, the director of the ICU at the Cleveland Clinic, and also talking with his friends in Europe. Throughout the Rio Grande valley there are three big groups of doctors that created a WhatsApp chat box so that they were talking to each other, sharing their findings and experiences every day. They agreed that so much misinformation was being promoted by the administration that they would chart their own path.

Then there was the issue of medications for his patients. In the beginning they did not have supplies of Remdesivir and had to wait weeks for it. The older members of their team used hydroxychloroquine out of desperation. Dr. Vallejo thought they were well intentioned, but should not have used it because there was no scientific basis for it. They began to use steroids in the early days because the coronavirus was such a significant inflammatory disease.

In August there were two new sources of support; the Department of Defense sent doctors that would take over one floor in the hospital. Then the hospital was able to bring over health care workers from other states, and three more ICUs were created in the hospitals. There was a neonatal unit that was as large as an airport hanger where they sent almost 50 patients, and they opened another floor at the MacAllen hospital. It was extremely difficult to get more doctors and nurses because there were not a sufficient number of them. Then there were doctors as well as a nurse practitioner who decided to retire because they couldn't handle the stress.

In fact a number of them throughout the country moved to New Zealand to work where thanks to their prime minister, Jacinda Ardern, they had a very low number of coronavirus patients, and there is universal health care where science is respected not criticized. They left our country because they did not have enough PPEs, and the lack of a coordinated response made them feel unsafe during the pandemic. Also medical practices closed during the pandemic according a survey by the Physicians Foundation, a non-profit group. Around 16,000 practices closed, some of them decided to change jobs, planned to retire early, or worried about their health because of their age or their medical conditions. Others stopped practicing during the surges and didn't feel able to resume their work or needed a break from the emotional toll of dealing with so many deaths. For example an anesthesiologist decided to quit after intubating seriously ill patients, worrying about his own health.[1] People don't realize how many physicians and nurses are infected by their patients. Throughout the country urgent care practices have replaced visits to internal medicine physicians, and pediatricians because they are afraid of catching the disease, and will only perform yearly wellness checks.

Another big issue for physicians are law suits against them. In Texas they have a tort reform, but Dr. Vallejo is very concerned about being sued again. He was sued once, but was cleared, and he concluded that lawyers are just trying to make money. The doctors were still learning about the disease every day, and deciding which medications to use. But Doctor Vallejo also had to deal with doctors that try out what he calls "miracle treatments," such as hydroxychloroquine as well as tea with aspirin and lemon. Someone came to the hospital with a vial extract of bovine spleen telling him that it was a cure for his family, and that if he didn't use it, he was going to sue him. An Australian paper wrote about another cure ivermectine that was in a petri dish, and very controversial yet a country in Latin America is buying a great deal of it. A doctor in Florida decided to use it, and published an unconvincing article on it in one of the important journals in pulmonary medicine, The Chest Journal. Dr. Vallejo found it dangerous that they had to spend so much money on refuting such papers. Everyday physicians have to read journals, and also the newspapers which became an arduous task during the pandemic.

As a doctor in the ICU, Dr. Vallejo is used to saving lives, not facing so many patients that die. With the pandemic he intubated patients, dealt with a patient's low blood pressure, sending patients to the Heart Hospital when they have high blood pressure, and helps people that are on the brink of death. In the first week of November when there was a third surge, he was having five deaths a day, and had never signed so many death certificates in a month. Then he was dealing with the fact that the patients' families were not there, and he was hearing screams on FaceTime when he had to give the terrible news of a patient's death. He found it emotionally and mentally overwhelming, and feels that he has some degree of PTSD (post traumatic stress disorder).

In the early months, he had a conversation with his wife, suggesting that they move to Costa Rica where he would practice telemedicine instead of being constantly exposed to the coronavirus in order to have a better lifestyle. He wanted to isolate himself instead of dealing with so much death and dying. He was overwhelmed by talking about comfort care, changing his patients' care to do not resuscitate, so they didn't have to give them chest compression. Then when he knew that there was no life expectancy, the only option just meant prolonging their suffering, which are such heart wrenching decisions. He remembers one horrible week when he had three patients who were talking to him, but he knew that they were very ill and were starting to deteriorate. By the end of the week, all three of them were dead, and one of them was 42 years old, the same age as him. The doctors did all that they could, giving them steroids, Remdesivir, convalescent plasma, and significant life support.

Then he went to a long-term acute care for people that are hospitalized for a long time who will have some sort of rehabilitation. But there was a also a time when people were very sick with respiratory failure, were intubated, had a tracheotomy, and were in good enough shape so that he could remove it, closing the hole in their necks. They were able to speak and that lifted his spirits. However many of his patients returned because being on severe ventilation for months leaves scars in their lungs. It helps to keep patients alive, but carries the risk of inflammation in the lungs becoming permanent, resulting in pulmonary fibrosis that lasts for a lifetime.

He found that people who return to the hospital finally began showing some empathy and wearing masks. He knew that so many states in our country do not require people to wear masks or impose lockdowns, and is deeply upset that science became politicized in our country. When he left the hospital at the end of the day, driving to an empty home, he drove past a restaurant that was packed with people, a sight that made him extremely angry. He has found that people like to think that they are not vulnerable, but views their version of freedom as irresponsibility. There has been a loss of the sense of community in our country that is so polarized with some states requiring masks and social distancing, and some refusing. Also there was a lack of leadership from the previous administration that would have informed people, and prevented them from attending large social gatherings, requiring masks and social distancing.

People travel from one state to another especially when they live near the border which results in a huge rise in cases because one state has issued requirements for masks and distancing while the other has not. People are tired of lockdowns, and want to enjoy themselves, not understanding how serious this pandemic is. As a result they gather in crowds for music festivals and restaurants.

The editorial board of the New England Journal of Medicine wrote articles that disapproved of the response to the coronavirus by the previous administration as did most of the physicians around the country. Dr. Vallejo is deeply upset by what he sees as a lack of empathy, and has worked hard to restore it himself. He has given thirty radio and press interviews nationally and locally, and never turned down an opportunity to talk with reporters such as the Wall Street Journal about this terrible illness. He also gave television interviews both nationally on CNN and on the BBC.

What really upset him is how President Trump was so cavalier about the pandemic, and how he touted racism. He saw the elections as based on hatred, and undermining our Democracy. As a result not only have the H1-B vises been terminated but also the J-1 visas, creating a shortage of doctors in our aging population.

He also started using TikTok to write about the coronavirus, and how he responds to it in order to educate people such as the importance of wearing a mask and social distancing. He had 55,000 followers in one day, and they respect him. He even criticized the former administration's response to this serious illness. He does it in English and Spanish because he found that Hispanics are lacking important information. He had wonderful responses compared to what was happening on social media claiming that everything is fine, that the coronavirus is part of a conspiracy, and promoting rallies without a mask. What really irritates him about the media is that it makes wearing a mask a weakness. He reached out despite his trying schedule, because despite his early response of wanting to move to another country, he loves doing this extra work and helping people in his community.

He is so pleased that followers that his TikTok have grown to 120,000, and to be able to educate people about the pandemic. On the one hand it helped him realize how poorly educated people are in this country that gave him another goal. On the other he responds to physicians and nurses who ask him about so many medications that should never be used on Covid-19 patients. In response he is able to give them scientific explanations as well. Given his many hours with TikTok followers for free, he sees it as a win- win project. The fact that he has reached out, and given so much of his time makes him happy about the results. Not many people realize that giving of oneself to make the world a better place is a source of deep satisfaction, and contentment. His parents have taught him how to be a good person, how to help people, and to think about other people, not just about himself. But given the toll of the pandemic he also found that he needed to engage in humorous activities, and even to laugh at himself to stay in good shape mentally and emotionally.

Dr. Vallejo has found TikTok to be very useful in other ways because he is up to date on vaccines, on therapeutics, and the monoclonal antibodies that fight the coronavirus. There has always been a disconnect in evaluating his patients because some of them with co-morbidities have done well while young people who have no illnesses do not do well. He found that a doctor has to be constantly learning about this illness, and read more in one year than in his whole career in medicine. His use of TikTok has created a wide response. For example, a person who was moving his family's furniture called out to him, "You are Dr. Vallejo, I know you from TikTok and learned so much from you."

He also created 30-second videos. They had such a large audience that he received responses from Peru, Venezuela, and Columbia, and has given radio interviews in Guadalajara, Jalisco. Although people have called him a hero, he doesn't feel like one. Rather, he feels that he is using his life well, and is an example for his children because they follow him, and learn so much from what he is saying. By his facial expressions they also know what kind of a day he experienced. He faces hate comments as well on the social media, but turns them around and uses them to teach people.

In fact he was offered an important academic position at the University of Massachusetts, but decided that he wanted to continue practicing close of Mexico because some of his family members live there, and he also wanted to help Hispanic people. The county he lives in is extremely poor, and he is concerned about the connection between poverty, and so many health problems such as obesity, hypertension, and asthma which make them more vulnerable to the coronavirus. He knew that these patients were not going to do well, and for many of them it was the first time they had ever seen a doctor. Because they worked in low paying jobs, they couldn't afford health insurance, and weren't allowed to take time off when they for an illness, unaware that they could get a coronavirus test for free or that they are legally entitled to paid sick leave if they contracted the virus. Forty percent of the people in the hospitals where he works do not have health insurance. Dr. Vallejo knows that Canada, and Western European countries have universal health care, and that their taxation system is more equitable.

The racial divide exists throughout our country. The Hispanic community, black Americans, and Native Americans contract the virus at a much higher degree than their white counterparts, and are four times more likely to be hospitalized by it. Doctors and scientists who keep track of the number of cases and death tolls are horrified, and many worry that the gap is greater than what the available data reveals. These groups are making their living in essential jobs in transit, nursing homes, living in crowded housing, and also in places that are highly polluted.

A population health specialist at the Mount Sinai Medical Center in New York commented that the cause of this is institutional racism, and added that race has been ignored in medicine which means that physicians don't collect that information or assess their performance on it. He also noted that the CDC research on it is very incomplete. Further there were no worker protections put in place when the nation began its lockdown phase. The Occupational Safety and Health issued guidelines such as wearing masks, social distancing and infection control programs advised by the CDC Federal agencies let the states to make rules, and the states left it to the employers. It is widely known that people who work low pay jobs do not receive the protections that they need for masks and social distancing.[2] At the end of the day Dr. Vallejo was telling people that they shouldn't go to work if they can't. But they need to feed their families and themselves so the only thing he can tell them is to wear a mask.

This is a disease that strikes Dr. Vallejo personally because of the poverty of his county. He also knows a teacher who was infected, a friend, and a friend of that friend, and the father of a friend because so many people in his community came down with the coronavirus. There was even a doctor who is a friend of his that became very ill. Hispanic families are very close, but his parents and his brother are in Mexico, and he hasn't been able to see them or even his sister who lives in Austin, Texas. But the closeness of Hispanic families means that they gather together for celebrations such as Mother's Day, birthdays parties, events which can make them vulnerable to infection.

The November surge was exacerbated by widespread travel when, over six million people wanted to join their families for the Thanksgiving holiday. Dr. Vallejo's county was seeing nearly 1,000 patients, but the health administration was prepared, and unlike many hospitals around the country they had enough ICU equipment. Dr. Vallejo is on the Medical Security Committee, a system that gives immediate responses to requests and complaints.

Staffing is still a big issue at the hospitals where he works and throughout Texas. They are overworked and overwhelmed by the number of patients that has inspired Dr. Vallejo to call, collaborate and share stories in El Paso, and Houston to learn how they are responding to the surge. They discuss myocardial conditions, and asymptomatic patients who are unaware that they have the coronavirus, but will suffer from it later on. They lost many good nurses during the pandemic because traveling nurses make three times the salary that their nurses earn. He feels that we need to pay them well, and provide them with PPEs.

El Paso was overwhelmed by the coronavirus in late November 2020 as inmates were paid to move hundreds of bodies into mobile morgues before the National Guards took over this painful task. Funeral homes turned storage closets into freezers to hold the bodies. Also, a crematorium was overused. Even chapels were overburdened. For those not on the frontlines of the virus; denial, boredom, and fear of losing their jobs divided the state. What makes it so sad is that there was a terrible event when a gunman killed 22 people and injured 24 outside of

Walmart. Everyone came together, and supported each other by putting up Mexican and American flags, with prayer circles coming together, flower arrangements, outdoor concerts, creating a deep feeling of community. Unfortunately when the coronavirus cases soared there were partisan recriminations between a Democrat who was a country judge, and a Republican who was a mayor, with the Democrat wanting a lockdown, and the Republican concerned about the effects on small businesses and the economy, both of which are at risk.

In so many counties in Texas, there are people going back and forth across the border with Mexico, to be with friends and families. But the racism that flared in the past years has affected Dr. Vallejo. At times, he found himself discriminated against because of his accent. For example when he answers a Page about returning a patient to the hospital, the reply is too often "I can't speak Spanish, let me get someone that can talk to you." However he is proud of his ancestry and his country. He likes to remind people that Texas, Arizona and New Mexico were previously part of Mexico, telling people, "it's not as if we crossed the border, the border crossed us." It would create important changes if people noticed that the names of so many physicians, and other professionals revealing that they or their families were immigrants.

Our population that hasn't suffered from the coronavirus have no idea of how physicians like Dr. Vallejo work long and difficult hours to help his patients, and that even though he worked so many hours, he spent his time educating people. He accomplished so much while the previous administration was claiming that all was well. Physicians do not watch regular television shows or spend hours on FaceTime. They spend very long and demanding days caring for the very ill, and dying in a place where they could become infected with the coronavirus, giving their expertise and lives to help our country.

After The Third Surge, Spring 2021.

In February 2021, a heavy snowstorm eliminated power in most of Texas that overwhelmed the power grid leaving many patients who were at home with the coronavirus losing heat and power and putting their lives at risk. They suffered from a loss of heat and electricity ending their portable oxygen supply. At the peak of the outages, near 4.5 million homes and business lost their power due to the ERCOT (Electric Reliability Council of Texas) that ignored warnings about the danger to its electricity. Doctors noted that when patients with serious respiratory conditions spend days without supplemental oxygen it affects their heart and lungs, with frigid conditions complicating breathing conditions leading to lung spasms.[3] Many of them went to emergency rooms, filling up crowded hospitals. However in order to reduce strain on hospitals' limited resources during the pandemic it became standard practice for hospitals to send most Covid-19 survivors home before they lungs had fully recovered. In short, it was a medical disaster.[4]

Luckily, the Rio Grande Valley only lost power for two days. In April 2021, Dr. Vallejo's had only 25 percent of his patients with the coronavirus as opposed to the 100 percent he saw last year. Now he can work in his office that was closed as well as the ICU seeing only 30 patients a day. He is caring for post Covid-19 patients in his outpatient clinic who are 50 percent of his patients, and whose problems will last for many years. Their problems are severe, and include tachycardia, dizziness, pulmonary fibrosis, a time to think about lung transplants. Covid-19 inflammation takes many months to heal, and he has to treat them as asthmatics. They are also experiencing mental fogginess due to micro-cells in the brain that block their circulatory system. He has also worked with patients with strokes, and pulmonary embolism giving them carbides arrhythmia. Some of them lose their hair, have clots in their lower extremities, chronic cough and chronic pain. He is upset that people are minimizing what is happening, and just focusing on the death rate going down although it is now more than half a million. He sees that as a simplistic view, and that we will have to deal with these issues for many years.

He is upset that we are not prepared for long term issues such as these. Then there are stigmas of people who were ill with the coronavirus as being dangerous, some of them reacting as if it were leprosy. Some of them are not being taken care of by their families, friends or even doctors. Although there are online groups where their issues are being discussed, it still leaves them on the margins without concern, sympathy or a willingness to talk about it.

In March, Governor Abbott lifted a statewide mask mandate because he said that it was an individual's decision. He also, opened up the economy including restaurants, stores, schools and malls without any limitations. He claimed that the pandemic was over while experts warned that reopening could result in a new surge. Even while Texas is giving vaccines to all adults, he insisted that they are voluntary. Then he claimed that they had reached herd immunity when only 19 percent of adults were vaccinated. The governor also issued an executive order banning government mandated vaccine passports.[4] Even President Biden has been very reticent about vaccine passports. Prominent Republicans like Governor Ron DeSantis, Mike Pompeo and Donald Trump jr. have denounced it although it is used in other places in the world. Now only some supermarkets are asking people to wear masks. Then there was the Spring break where a few thousands college students gathered at the Saint Padre Island by the beach shouting and screaming without wearing masks or social distancing. That happened in Florida too, but the police went after them.

Dr. Vallejo is also concerned about insufficient testing in the U.S. In an article in the Wall Street Journal, a professor at John Hopkins University pointed out that we only catch 20 to 25 percent with our testing because it is very dependent on the timing of the test. Also, a lot of people are asymptomatic, but they don't get tested. There are people with very low symptoms who refuse to get tested because they don't think it is necessary but who nevertheless can spread the coronavirus.

He is also upset because in the U.S. we often refer to the immigrants waiting at our Southern border as spreaders of Covid-19. People don't realize that they are refugees, fleeing danger, drought, and gangs that are killing family members regularly. They are not coming to make money or to have the dream of a good life since that is gone for most immigrants. They work extremely hard, live in poverty, and hope that the second or third generation will have a better life. If they are a woman or a child there is a good chance that they would get raped or molested. Not many people realize that the border guards under the previous administration also raped women and girls or that immigrants made to stay in Mexico are physically abused. Dr. Vallejo wants them to be treated in a humane way because when people refer to them as a crisis on the border it makes them seem as if they will create havoc in our country. Unfortunately the number of immigrants also feeds into the White Supremacy movement, and far too many people use them as scapegoats. In fact, many of the people involved in the insurrection of January 6 came from towns where that were against immigrants and minorities.[5]

Dr. Vallejo is still spending a great deal of time on informing people about the coronavirus. He is still on TikTok and now has 307,000 followers. He has removed his personal page from Facebook in exchange for a professional page under Dr. Federico Vallejo, and has around 11,000 followers. He also uses Instagram where he has 8,000. Then he has interviews with the local media to talk about the fourth wave of the surge, and was featured on CNN, The Wall Street Journal, the BBC. He regularly appears on Spanish Univision, Telemondo, a platform in Mexico, a radio program in Columbia, and a Television station in Paraguay. Not many people realized how high the number of variants were in both the U.S. and Latin America. Brazil's lack of care had resulted in the coronavirus spilling over in other countries such as Paraguay, Peru and Argentina. In Texas, the B.1.1.7 has risen to almost 75 percent and is wreaking havoc in continental Europe while rising exponentially in the U.S.

What hurts Dr. Vallejo the most now is not the pandemic, but widespread misinformation. The anti-vaccine movement comes from 12 different sources. In fact millions on social media proclaim that the vaccine causes death, and he wonders why lies are being allowed on the social media. In fact the Supreme Court overturned a lower court opinion that President Trump could not block critics from Twitter. But when he lost the election Twitter canceled his account. Judge Clarence Thomas said that the real work for the government might be to limit the ability of social media companies to remove users.[6] Dr. Vallejo sees that the strategy of keeping people uninformed helps those in power. Part of that misinformation is twofold, how our educational system is much less demanding than it was for more than a decade, that only 24 percent of our population read newspapers, and the rest are not eager to spend the time to be fully informed.

There are also a great number of healthcare workers in nursing homes that refuse to be vaccinated. It is a difficult and complex issue that involves ethics, law, labor relations, and ingrained American values. The CDC and OSHA have been silent on the issue while state and local governments have a long history of requiring vaccinations for schoolchildren. The EEOC (Equal Employment Opportunity Commission) concluded that employers could exclude an employee from the workplace for refusing to be vaccinated. However the worker must be offered telework or be placed on leave, as well as be given exemptions when a vaccination would conflict with his religious belief. According to the Washington Post-Kaiser Family Foundation, a poll revealed that six in ten people would support a coronavirus vaccine and four in ten would oppose it.[7]

Dr. Vallejo is continuing to work long hours on the pandemic, but he sees his efforts in three ways; the disease, misinformation about vaccines or miracle cures, and the lack of empathy. He is very concerned that we are focusing on freedom and privacy which he regards as a way of spreading the disease in an anonymous way so the person involved doesn't have to deal with the consequences. For example when he had finished with a patient in his office, he told him that he should get a coronavirus vaccine. The patient declined telling him that both the pastor and a doctor in his congregation told him that he shouldn't get it. Dr. Vallejo suggested that in that case he should see another doctor he will find for him or the doctor in his congregation that told him not to get vaccinated because he didn't want to expose his staff. Dr. Vallejo is passionate about the truth and finds that people are used to lies because they are easy responses to a very difficult and complex situation. Too many of us have not embraced a shared sense of identity, and responsibility for each other that could delay the end of the pandemic.

DR. SUSAN LY

The Beginning of the Pandemic

Dr. Susan Ly was eager to become an emergency room physician because she wanted to do something that would help people. She knew that she could diagnose certain conditions, and if not she would know where they could receive help, something she found very gratifying. But everything changed when she first started hearing about the coronavirus in January and February 2020, that was the result of cases from Wuhan, China when people came to the state of Washington and MA. Their first patients were being monitored in early March to mid-March, but they didn't have tests available yet so they were examining symptoms.

The issue across most hospitals around the country including areas where so many patients arrived was the need for PPEs, that the required volume of that equipment wasn't available. They weren't able to provide it because there are certain types of stockpiles available for such situations, such as biological or chemical disasters, medication antidotes that includes PPEs and N95s. Fortunately her hospital soon had that much needed equipment. But for a while they had to go by protocols so if a staff member didn't have certain equipment, they could use something else. However she has friends in another hospital who didn't have access to that gear, were ready to receive a shipment for the staff when all of a sudden it was rerouted to Washington D.C. and redistributed. Then there were some hospitals where the staff had to use trash bags to protect themselves.

In those early days, they were nervous because people were coming to the ER with severe problems who would also be vomiting or have nausea. The staff had no idea if those would be symptoms of the coronavirus. They wondered if was just a respiratory virus, or a symptom of something less severe such as the flu. There were so many unknowns, and of course that included treatment, but physicians looked for signs of any complications that could make the patients hospitalized. The only recourse they had at the time was to say, "Go home, good luck, and if you get sicker, come back in." That was a scary moment for doctors on the frontlines. They didn't feel that they could do anything for their patients, and didn't know anything about a possible treatment. She felt as if she were on a drowning ship and that she couldn't get enough life jackets to help them.

According to Dr. Ly in the months of June and July 2020, she found that the U.S. benefited from being one of the last countries to have the virus. European and Asian countries were using medications with different regiments to handle it, as well as data revealing which medications were the most successful. She saw that as an amazing feat of science because of how quickly the studies resulted in diagnosis and medications. She always had such a large and diverse population in her unit, patients of all ages with different ethnicities, genders, and diverse risk factors, and was so concerned.

However, what usually takes years, only took months to discover what really works. Even when our country was at a loss, China and Asia had a good grasp of the situation, and had better containment than the U.S although our government ended our cooperation with China in the early days of the breakout. Italy's hospitals were very crowded, but they were able to deal with the outbreak. In the late Fall, our country started to see that steroids were a benefit in certain populations thanks to their use in Britain.

She felt that her training has helped, but that her work was amplified to a new level. Nevertheless she is thankful to have a strong support system at home, something that not every healthcare provider has. Her parents live only thirty minutes away from her, and her husband is working at home. At that time although she was worried and frightened by the coronavirus, she felt that she had the support of the community, and that everyone was rooting for her, wishing her good luck. They also had time to take care of their staff, and came up with protocols for the hospital. Dr. Susan Ly was part of a committee that decided how to respond if a patient arrived with the symptoms of the virus, and how to handle that on the floor of the ICU.

Dr. Ly found herself with two goals, taking care of her patients, and learning at the same time. She was very worried about the coronavirus, and how it was spreading at a time when she didn't have the information she needed. In the early months patients were coming in with other illnesses such as strokes and infections. Then they were starting to see links between these illnesses, and she asked herself why they were coming in with strokes and blood clots, and also had the coronavirus infection. Learning on the fly with illnesses that she didn't understand or had a full knowledge of was not how she was taught medicine. Then she saw patients with so many months of symptoms. It was hard to know how long it was going to last for the patients she treated. She wondered if it was going to take a lifetime or whether they had a risk of more deterioration.

Over the year, people who had the proper treatment for the infection, and who may have spent months intubated, were well enough to be released. But once at home they would have difficulty breathing, and a fatigue that changed their lives, or they were seeing other physicians for severe problems in their organs.

She remembers when Ebola was a big scare at the time when they had new cases, and was terrified because she knew how deadly it was, but there was an understanding of its symptoms. They knew more about vaccines, and were able to quickly contain it. Yet in December 2020, a new variant of the coronavirus was discovered that spreads more rapidly doubling roughly every 10 days, potentially bringing a surge of new cases, and an increased risk of death. The variant appeared a number of times as a result of people traveling from Britain to the U.S. over Thanksgiving and Christmas, although in MA, people were required to show negative results of testing at the time of their arrival. The mutation B.1.1.7. is 30 to 40 percent higher than then more common variants, potentially bringing a surge of new cases and an increased risk of death.[1]

There are also mutations in Brazil, P.1, and South Africa, B.1.351, that have appeared in the U.S. Another one called E484K and given the nickname of EeK, has appeared in the three variants. All viruses mutate, and scientists have said that these variants have not changed our understanding of their transmission or impacted the necessity of getting vaccinated. They have assured physicians that the vaccines still offer protection. An epidemiologist at the John Hopkins Center for Health spoke about the necessity of disease prevention such as vaccines, social distancing, masks, contact tracing, isolation and quarantine that are essential for reducing the spread of the coronavirus.[2] There was a countrywide need for testing and contact tracing as well. There were some efforts such as home testing underway, but not enough.

Since the previous administration left the response to the coronavirus up to each state, there was no uniform response to prevention with a number of states such as Ohio, Michigan, Texas and Mississippi opening up restaurants, group gatherings, and not requiring masks or social distancing.

Then there is an anti-vaccine movement as well as the anti-vax movements that have appeared on Facebook, a critical organizing tool. Its social networking services can lead to more confrontational tactics by groups committed to false ideas. They placed videos on a site that complains about "discrimination" and "medical tyranny," asserting that the masks restrict breathing, and that the Constitution forbids requiring their use. Part of the extreme right, these groups accuse the "elites" for enriching themselves by creating the coronavirus, and the vaccine. And they have been active. For example, in Los Angeles, health authorities have been administering shots to 8,000 people a day at Dodger Stadium when a protest by these groups forced authorities to close the stadium gates delaying thousands of motorists lined up to receive vaccinations. While doctors are rushing to vaccinate as many people as possible to outpace the variant, such protests came at a critical time.[3]

However, when vaccines were being publicized and becoming available, a large part of our population was anxious to get them. The new administration established sites where our minorities and impoverished could be vaccinated, and hoped to have the whole country vaccinated by the end of the summer 2021. The Biden administration invoked the Defense Production Act to increase supplies, and drew upon the federal resources to increase the number of vaccination sites. For example the administration set up three mass vaccination centers in Arlington, Dallas, and Huston, plus two centers in Brooklyn and Queens. Eventually, President Biden publicized the fact that he had enough vaccines for every adult by the end of May 2021.

Dr. Ly sees the coronavirus as covert and dangerous, with asymptomatic patients, and those who died from it. The severity range is a combination that has not been seen in a pandemic virus. Also, the testing that is in process is not happening everywhere, and the actual number of infections is much higher. An infections disease expert at Columbia University found that disparity with 919 infections out of 100,000 tested, and 998 asymptomatic out of 100,000. [4]

A Physical and Emotional Toll

Dr. Ly is experiencing a huge physical and emotional toll. She found that some staff members are so fatigued, and even stopped caring because they were involved in working with coronavirus patients for too long. The New England Journal of Medicine described the psychological trauma of health care workers as a parallel pandemic.[5] Unfortunately the general public has stopped thinking about health care workers, and are unaware of the consequences of their work. While in the early months, healthcare workers' communities celebrated the medical staff, in the winter months of 2021 they were feeling crushed and unappreciated.

What made this even more stressful for doctors like Susan Ly was the lack of leadership in the previous administration, while countries like New Zealand and Japan responded to the outbreak at the very beginning with a number of policies to contain it. President Trump was refusing to listen to any evidence based research, or to public health advisors like Dr. Anthony Fauci and Dr. Deborah Brix. He also ended our membership in the WHO that always had a good opinion of the U.S. She found that the result of a lack of attention, blaming the states, and referring to the coronavirus on racist terms set us back. That also provoked widespread violence against Asian Americans that led to thousands of deaths as well as verbal and physical assaults.

She also found that our response was so poor on so many different levels, and discovered that people don't want complex news, but simple ones like the stories on Fox News. And so many people are thinking that the government is controlling us because they didn't send the message about wearing masks and social distancing before. Dr. Ly sees these views as dangerous, and also that people who are hospitalized or who have died are just someone in the news. That means that the coronavirus is not part of our conversations, and people are unaware of the trauma our health care workers' experience or do not seem to care as they go about their daily lives.

Then there is the social media that far right groups use to discredit the pandemic, and people who were working to control it. For example, there were detailed plans by a right wing group to kidnap the governor of Michigan, Gretchen Whitmer, because of anger over her coronavirus measures. They were meeting repeatedly for firearms training, plus practicing to build explosives until they were caught by the FBI. With just newspapers, it was easier to control misinformation. Investigative journalism is very important to preserve our democracy. However, nationwide 2000 local newspapers have closed, and half of all newsroom jobs have been eliminated, something that accelerated during the pandemic. Facebook and Google received billions in revenue while local newspapers are having difficulty raising money for advertisements.[6]

In an age of social media it's more than difficult to control the spread of disinformation that becomes truth to people. It has divided our country with friends and family members no longer speaking to each other, and display a strong need to be right. The noted journalist Nicholas Kristof who visited Oregon where he grew up on a farm, found himself talking to so many people about what was really happening when they came up to him to complain. He found that listening to people with opposing views was helpful. It relieved their anxiety. He was able to do so because he grew up there. Social media has become like a game, and is also an addiction. For example, a professor had to tell his students to stop using their iPhones during his class.

Now many millions are drawn to extremist groups on Telegram and Signal where far right, and criminal groups create their own version of reality. Conspiracy groups like QAnon were used to delay coronavirus efforts, and one Congresswoman, Marjorie Taylor Greene has promoted it. Millions of people are drawn to extremist views not because they are convinced by the facts, but rather that it gives them a sense of purpose, of belonging, and filling the void in their lives. It is not only a matter of public safety, but should also be viewed as a health issue by reaching out to them with caring messages of mental health and mindfulness. These groups also appeal to people who see our society as uncaring, distrust authority, and are angry at the growing inequality between rich and poor that has been exacerbated by the pandemic. Dr. Susan Ly has been very concerned about having preventive medicine that she sees as an important route to health.

Her children are five and seven year old, and she is trying to raise them in a world where social media is dominant, and so many people are trying to get information electronically. She regrets that we are no longer in a time when people have to look things up for information, but just go to Google or Alexa, and the answers will be provided. There is no emphasis on trying to discover things or to engage in learning that is a process used throughout a person's life. Politicians and even people who write opinion columns in the news use twitter as well as people who enjoy spreading their news. It makes them feel powerful and important. Our culture is inundated with social media.

PBS made a documentary on the creation of the radio in the U.S. It showed people glued to the radio, listening and believing what they heard. Even though initially it reached a small part of our population compared to today; comedy, soap operas and news were aired, even President Roosevelt gave weekly speeches. Now there are right wing radio shows that once featured Rush Limbaugh, and currently include Glenn Beck and Mark Levin. Since they are dependent on corporate paychecks, they are not as rabid. However, social media is available every moment of the day and can be transported. A professor of doctoral students found her students complaining about having to read books, preferring to get their information on the web. An important part of learning that is disappearing is taking the necessary time and effort as well as exploring different ways of thinking. Dr. Susan Ly has read stories to her children and remembers a time when books were a source of entertainment with families sitting in one room, and reading books together.

What has also changed during the pandemic is the behavior of people in Emergency Rooms and even ICU's. She has patients come in with all of the classic symptoms of the coronavirus, shortness of breath and fever. They were surprised when she told them that they were infected with the coronavirus, and that they should have taken the measures they need to

keep them healthy. Like so many other doctors, she found that some
patients didn't believe that they were ill with the coronavirus. She reads
the New England Journal of Medicine that is the most prestigious
medical journal, and saw an editorial about how unsuccessful our
leadership was during the Trump administration. It detailed how that
administration drove the pandemic to become the country with the
largest number of infections and deaths in the world. This was before
India became overwhelmed with it in the spring of 2021, and had the
most deaths a day of any country. At a time when science was
undermined and politicized in the U.S. there were voices of truth, but so
many of us live in the present, and are unaware how it was silenced
throughout history in so many places in the world. The fact that the
journal felt that it had to take a stance says a lot about what was
happening in 2020.

It's important to remember the reaction about seat belts. People railed
against using them, but the younger generation was more resilient. Their
teachers told them to wear them to ensure their safety, and they
persuaded their parents. Dr. Ly doesn't see any children fighting over
masks and social distancing although it was hard for them. She believes
that the younger generation will accept, and move forward to do the right
thing, and sees them as more resilient than adults.

Many people are finding both inconvenient. Dr. Ly thinks that if an
everyday convenience is all that they are facing they should consider
themselves lucky. She sees us as a "me society", that we have lost our
sense of community, that we have defined freedom as meaning that we
can do anything we want regardless of the consequences. Unfortunately
so many people see efforts to follow the protocols for safety as an
impingement on their freedom. For example, one woman complained
because she had to pick up an order from a retail store outside of the
entrance. Meanwhile there is another version of freedom. There are so
many refugees and immigrants who are fleeing war and violence in their
countries while we are against admitting them, thinking that they are
criminals, and also will take our jobs.

In the winter of 2021, Dr. Susan Ly was seeing an escalation of
respiratory illnesses, with patients who are much sicker; with heart

attacks, strokes, acute asthma, all of which are coronavirus complications. But now she found that there was not enough space to hold her patients, or visitors in the waiting room. She was surrounded by chaos with patients yelling at her because they have no visitor policy except for minors. She found that it was like people going into a store, and refusing to wear a mask when they are required to. Families were angry, telling her that they couldn't understand why they couldn't come in. She replied that they are doing this to avoid the risk to them, the patients and the staff. She worried about how crowded it was, that there were patients who watched people having a stroke or a heart attack, and yet were making a fuss because they didn't receive a blanket or had help from a nurse even though they had been there for less than a half-hour.

Although they know how to deal with their coronavirus patients that are very ill, Dr. Susan Ly has to deal with new issues that was more stressful. They have patients who have had the virus for six months yet were unable to see their doctor because his or her office was inundated. There are so many primary care doctors that didn't want to see them because they didn't feel comfortable, and told them that they have to go to ED (Emergency Department) that is a boarding area for patients awaiting admission to the ER.

According to data collected by the MACEP (The Massachusetts College of Emergency Physicians), people suffering from a mental health crisis go to the ER for help, but unfortunately there are not enough beds for them in psychiatric units. Because of the pandemic, hospitals had fewer available beds, and they had to reserve some of them for isolation if they tested possible for the coronavirus. There were more people suffering from increased depression and anxiety coming in because mental health issues were exacerbated by the pandemic. The head of the MACEP has seen a big increase in patients waiting for inpatient beds in psychiatric units, but also for medical conditions.[7] Dr. Ly has seen the increase in psychiatric patients that were suffering, and unable to get the help that they need. She has found that talking to a psychiatrist over the telephone is not going to solve the isolation, and the anxiety that young people are experiencing.

For a growing number of teenagers a year of social isolation led to suicidal thinking and behavior that rose by 47 percent, many of them emotionally sensitive. They face so many new stresses because of fewer social interactions at a time when they are growing in so many ways, and they need to be a part of the community. Because many of them could longer engage in sports or were unable to spend time with their peer groups they felt a loss of their identity.[8] Also, there are not many places that they could turn to for help other than the ER. For proper help they would need a psychiatric diagnosis, and in person therapy rather than lying in a hospital bed without knowing why they are waiting there or where they are going. They lost a predictable and normal life, and felt a kind of grief that is not recognized in our society.

In fact Dr. Susan Ly believes that everyone has a right to healthcare as do countries such as France and Italy. She would like healthcare to include mental health after what she has seen in the ER where there are so many people who have no health care and no insurance. She would like our country to have a preventive health care system so that people who have high blood pressure don't have to go to the ER with strokes or heart attacks. European countries that provide universal healthcare have high taxes, a policy that is difficult to promote in the U.S.

She also saw that psychological help was lacking in too many hospitals, although they do have peer systems like buddy systems. What many doctors and nurses need are respite, time off to rest and recover at a time when there aren't enough healthcare workers. She is also upset that the restrictions we need to avoid infection are not being enforced, and refers to it as "like a slap in the face." She could tell them how many sick patients she has seen and how many have died, but they are not interested unless they have known someone who is close to them who has been affected. She also wonders why it is so hard to make the public understand that this is a pandemic that affects real people and their lives. But she also understands the other side of the spectrum that we can't live in quarantine forever, and that you have to make decisions that are appropriate for you in some degree. There are going to be families that quarantine in a bubble, but they should try not to stray out of that.

Dr. Susan Ly understands that it is hard for our leadership to think about the economy and the pandemic at the same time, why Governor Baker lifted restrictions on restaurants and some small businesses in early March. However she saw some curfews lifted when the numbers of infections were going up. The same is true throughout many countries such as the UK when at first restaurants and bars were urged to stay open by Boris Johnson, and when there was a surge, he created a complete lockdown. People coming from abroad were forced to stay in a hotel at their own expense for 14 days of quarantine even if they have a home there.

Dealing with so many issues besides the overwhelming work at the ER is more than demanding and Dr. Susan Ly needs hope. When she goes into work she just thinks that every patient has the coronavirus because it is so prevalent in the community. She is being very methodical; wearing a surgical mask and eye goggles that make her feel secure. She wears an N95, and a respiratory cover every time she checks into work. She doesn't know if people who are homeless and intoxicated are infected or not, and they might refuse to wear masks, and talk back to her. This is a whole new stress that she has encountered in her career. Although she has support from her family and co-workers, many times she has sat in her car and cried before and after her shift. She does vent with her co-workers because other people do not understand the situation that she is in. She finds that it is important to find an outlet for such anxiety whether venting, crying or talking. She knows that things are not going to change quickly, and may continue for a long time. She sees people going on vacations, and still going to restaurants.

In fact she went to the presidential inauguration, but when she came back from D.C. no one checked her when she got off the plane although Massachusetts requires people coming from other states or abroad to have a document saying that they had been tested and were negative. She found that it's like an honor system. Some of her co-workers had a lay over in Georgia where the cases were high, and they were also not questioned when they returned.

Dr .Susan Ly knows what many people are unaware of, the death toll of our health workers. As of January 2021, 3,332 healthcare workers have died which does not include their family members. She and her co-workers have seen so many people die, and have been affected by it. Then there are families who have lost their beloved members. The second and third surge affected a lot of her staff who became infected with the coronavirus or their family members. And so many healthcare workers died in the line of duty, ER and ICU healthcare doctors and nurses. "It is like going to battle and seeing your brothers and sisters go down." She wonders if it could be her or one of her loved ones, that she could potentially bring home the coronavirus. That type of worry never goes away.

Unfortunately there is no federal government's plan to count the number of workers who are infected and have died. Studies have revealed that medical professionals make up 10 percent to 20 percent of all coronavirus cases in the early pandemic though they account for four percent of our population. The CDC relies on reporting from state health departments, and a least a dozen states do not participate in its reporting process. A researcher at the University of Michigan said that without complete data on the health of our medical workers it is not possible to come up with interventions.[9]

Then there are medical workers who have survived the coronavirus challenges yet can be plagued by fatigue, and impaired lung function. Doctors and nurses who have been health care professionals for many years are the most vulnerable. Some hospitals are so short staffed that they require their medical workers who have symptoms of the coronavirus to stay on their jobs.

It has been found that pandemic stress puts health care workers at an even higher risk of despair. One emergency room physician feels the anxiety of constant intubations, and PPE shortages. Then there are the quarantines, school closings, social isolation, and shelter in place orders that have changed the way we live. Frontline health workers in overwhelmed areas are exhausted and traumatized from treating patients with the coronavirus. Health care providers in all areas struggle to cope with the complicated politics that surround the pandemic, and the lack of a national strategic plan to deal with it.

Then there are doctors and nurses have committed suicide. A well known case is Dr. Lorna Breen an ER physician who committed suicide from the stress of witnessing so many deaths. Her brother in law Mr. Feist, and his wife who was Lorna Breen's sister started the Lorna Breen Heroes Foundation, a non-profit created to help the emotional well-being of health care workers. They worked with politicians and health care experts to develop the Lorna Breen Health Care Provider Protection Act in order to deal with mental and behavioral conditions, and suicide among health care professionals.[10] In the fall of 2020, polls of emergency physicians throughout the country found that 87 percent felt more stressed since the onset of the pandemic. Healthcare workers are dealing with the stress of seeing so many patients die, their own anxiety about themselves and their family members being infected. Fortunately a number of support groups for them have been created throughout the country, such as #/FirstRespondersFirst, at Harvard T.H. Chan School of Public Health.[11]

How Lives Have Changed for Children

Then there are the children around our country who are either unable to attend school or only do so two or three days a week. Dr. Susan Ly's children are in a hybrid system with her daughter in school three days a week, and her son in preschool two days a week. She feels fortunate because that makes up for being on screen for so much time. But her nieces and nephews who live in California are completely online. It is not easy for children of all ages learning remotely because they suffer from isolation while they are going through their formative years, and some of them become depressed. Children need to be with each other of the same age because it is an important part of their growth and exploration of their world.

Then there are young people who are learning on line in college which could be the best years of their lives, and who are unable to have a graduation ceremony which is such an important moment. Too many young adults feel as if their lives are on hold. Some of them are fortunate to have a job that is on line, but that doesn't deal with the loneliness they feel. There are many young people who don't have the money, and equipment they need to learn on line that is exacerbating the inequality in our society. When their schools were open they were below par. We need to focus on our at risk population. Also our society is hurting because too many of us miss family reunions. We don't think about families that live very far apart from each other or who live in different countries.

In February of 2021 the CDC announced that K-12 schools should be reopened as soon as possible, and offered a step by step plan to get students back into their classrooms and resolve the debate that is polarizing communities throughout the country. The recommendations were intended to respond to the disagreement about opening primary schools up to the eighth grade. The President prioritized opening schools, but was facing the new variants of the coronavirus. However the American Federation of teachers Unions thanked the CDC for clearer guidance, but the National Education Association argued that it's strategy would be difficult to enact without more federal funding. There is still disagreement among parents, and between political parties with the Republicans wanting schools to open full time. The consensus of experts goes against some school administrators, teachers' unions and parent groups. In large cities, teachers have threatened to strike if schools open even though they will be vaccinated by next fall. Both communities whose schools were open, and those that were closed believed that they made the right choice. In early March, President Biden announced his intention to vaccinate every teacher and gradually reopen schools.

Doctors found that limiting children's time in school could lead to depression, hunger, isolation and learning less. An emergency room physician found that she sees so many children in her unit that are experiencing mental distress. This toll has led a number of pediatricians to argue for reopening schools. In fact the CDC found that visits to the ER by adolescents for mental health increased by 31 percent during the period between March and October 2020, compared with the same months in the previous year. The March 2021 journal of the American Academy of Pediatrics found higher rates of children from 11 to 21 years old had a higher rate of wanting to commit suicide than in 2020.[12]

It is not surprising given that the coronavirus is so new, and that only in 2021 have medical experts been able to speak out. It is not comfortable for any group to deal with such enormous challenges. Also minority students live in the poorest most infected areas, and they are the ones who have experienced the greatest consequences of not being able to attend school.[13]

Changes in our Medical System

Dr. Susan Ly is not only concerned about having health care available to everyone who needs it, she is also upset about the changes in personnel in our medical system. There are many nurses who study for a Doctor of Nursing online which is an extension of the master's degree, the Doctor of Nursing Practice, the Clinical Nurse Leader, the Nurse Practitioner, and the Physician's Assistant. They were originally designated for healthcare leadership roles versus practice roles. She sees it as a problem because the general public doesn't know the difference, for example if you are going to see a doctor of nursing because they refer to themselves as doctors. She found that it confuses a whole spectrum such as a patient seeing someone who has a tenth of the education in time, knowledge, experience, and training as a medical doctor, what she sees as a quick fix that is detrimental to the health care system.

In Massachusetts, nurse practitioners can work independently on their own, providing easier access and is now the norm. Dr. Susan Ly knows patients whose primary care physician is a nurse practitioner who has no oversight. When they do work in the right field, and the right role she sees them as priceless. But she found that in roles that they were never intended for their jobs become twice as hard because all these consults send their patients to the emergency room who don't need to be there. Then they get upset when they are billed for overwork, or when they have had excessive testing that was not necessary. She sees a need to improve the control of each role in healthcare so they can have a smoother streamlined system with uniform medical records that can be transferred from one hospital to another. Unfortunately, she can no longer communicate with primary care physicians in the same way that she used to.

Dr. Ly also knows that there are not enough physicians, that it is cheaper to hire a nurse practitioner than a doctor, that emergency room graduates are having a tough time finding their first full time job. They used to be constantly called by head hunters. Because we don't have enough physicians, they are now being replaced by an alternate work force that is less expensive. Neither political party is more concerned about skills rather than expense, one wanting to spend less on educating physicians, and the other preferring nurses who are educated into new roles. Some doctors have resigned as a result, and spend one day each week at urgent care centers.

We don't have sufficient physicians, but residency programs haven't kept up with the rising number of applications in recent years. In 2020, the Association of Medical Colleges released a finding that the U.S. would have to confront a greater shortage of doctors in the coming years that would triple the current 54,000. Hospitals sometimes use the Electronic Residency Application Service software program to filter out various applications. There are doctors who have graduated from medical school, and are left with thousands of dollars in student loans and default on debts. In addition to the need for the new medications and vaccines, there is a need to look at the whole picture.[14]

That picture includes a new phenomenon, businesses now wanting to buy medical groups such as Optum, a United Heath subsidiary. It is currently is in talks to acquire Atrius Health, a 715 physician group based in Newton, Massachusetts, according to the Boston Business Journal. Optum has signed a memorandum of understanding to acquire the non-profit Atrius. The proposed deal comes after Optum acquired Worcester, Mass-based Reliant Medical Group in April 2018. This is not an easy time for medical students and practices, because it will mean laying off doctors.

Dr. Susan Ly is facing a number of important and difficult issues. But she is dedicated to her job, intellectually and emotionally, at a fraught time in the pandemic. Not many people realize the extraordinary effort she has made while they are going about their daily lives. She should be celebrated by her many achievements, and for the important role she plays in our lives.

DR. EDY KIM

Science and Medicine

While we think of the doctors and nurses in critical care, not many people realize the many demands that are placed on the hospital's' operational structure, and personnel. Large hospitals may have several ICU's, and have to organize them differently. Thus many of them call back former physicians or lab technicians that have left for new jobs because they need more medical staff. Physicians found themselves managing new clinical care and medications, and doing triage during the pandemic's overflow.

Because Brigham and Women in Massachusetts is a research focused hospital, and the only medical ICU in the country, almost 90 percent of attending physicians spend more time in the laboratory. All them work for a couple of months in ICU, and then spend the rest of the time in the laboratory. Thus when they had the first coronavirus patient in March 2020, they also had a very knowledgeable group of attending doctors, especially during the surge. A lot of people who would usually come to the ICU in the first months didn't show up which Dr. Kim considered good for those with the coronavirus, but not for the those who needed immediate care, but were afraid of getting infected with the virus. That enabled the doctors to work with the high numbers of coronavirus patients. There were not enough nurses and respiratory therapists, but fortunately they had enough money to offer higher salaries to the traveling nurses. Also since elective surgery needs and the ambulatory volume were low, the nurses who worked there could be reassigned to ICU.

Dr. Kim has a Ph.D in science, and found it very difficult to be just a scientist who is not a physician. He does research on immunology, examines human samples that are hard to find, and has some clinical context that a non- physician would not have. His major occupation is in pulmonary fibrosis that is relevant to the coronavirus because it attacks the lungs, and he has also worked on cardiac issues, bringing a lot of insight to his work in the ICU.

What he found unique about coronavirus is that usually clinical guidelines are established over the years with a group of individuals gathering in a conference, and putting together a working group recommendation. With the arrival of the coronavirus he had to invent clinical guidelines in just a couple of days. Two of the things that helped at Brigham and Women's were that physicians with experience in the laboratories were available to invent structures based on their information, and in the ICU they had to make important choices for the doctors. The lab world and the ICU world was a good fit for the coronavirus.

For instance, they disapproved of the high flow nasal cannula. Dr. Kim found that many ICUs were using it very early. Since there is so much virus in a patient's nose, many nurses and respiratory therapists were afraid of catching the coronavirus. In the first wave, a lot of them didn't use high flow nasal cannula at all although they were used in Texas and other states. That led to some people being intubated. in June when they began using high flow cannula. They also knew that there were so many side effects of mechanical ventilation. When, a patient gets sedated sometimes for weeks they get delirious when they are taken off of the ventilator. They used intubation earlier than expected because people were worried about a chaotic situation in the ICU. However, after a week the anesthesiologists went back to their usual work. They never ran out of ventilators because the people in charge of securing them were able to purchase some, rent some, and acquire temporary travel ventilators used to take people to the MRI. They never ran out.

At their peak the hospital had about 105 patients intubated, and 100 more on the regular floor. The Massachusetts General Hospital had about 180. At Brigham and Women they usually had patients divided between ICU's, one for surgery, and one for cardiac illness. Before the coronavirus, the ICU had a maximum of 20 patients. Having 100 patients in an ICU with the coronavirus was overwhelming.

Because the coronavirus affects every organ, it was more than difficult, because everything that they took for granted became scarce. There is a special kind of dialysis, which needs a machine that works around the clock. They ran out of those machines, and had to use one for another patient every 10 hours. When they wanted to measure someone's blood oxygen levels, a lab test that requires a special type of syringe, there were not enough. As a result they had to send a message to their training doctors to only send off that test if it is really crucial, and to use the finger pulse option measurements as much as possible.

The beginning was difficult for him with so many patients, and so many decisions to make. The ICU chief in charge of the response to the coronavirus asked him to help them out, and he helped organize their clinical guidelines. In retrospect they should have done it on zoom. Instead they brought together a number of ICU physicians for three or four days to review what they learned about what was happening in China, Seattle, and Italy. They also shared knowledge about ARDS (acute respiratory distress syndrome), lung injuries, and motor accidents. With ARDS a patient get sick for a few weeks, heals, and then the body injures the lung, establishing a pattern. Unfortunately there are no medications for that condition, only placing patients on a ventilator, hoping that they would heal. They had debates about whether the ARDS is the same as any other sick patient in ICU, regardless of the cause. While the coronavirus has some similarities to ARDS patients, there is a lot that was unique about this new disease. They decided that the treatments for it would not be successful for ARDS patients. They are still discussing new information about this issue.

Dr. Kim found that some laboratory tests, clinical findings in ICU, and patient characteristics gave them hints on who would get better, and who would get worse. The good news was that they have some new treatments besides oxygen, anti-inflammatory drugs, and steroids. If people in ICU worsen, they now treat them with a second anti-inflammatory drug, one used for rheumatoid arthritis. It's a monoclonal antibody, but different from the Regeneron that President Trump was given. Rheumatoid arthritis patients' have their immune system attack their joints, and are given monoclonal antibodies that specifically targets the immune pathway. The physicians-scientists have discovered that the immune system of the coronavirus quickly declines.

They carried out a clinical trial in January 2021, and found that if people came into the ICU with the coronavirus they should give them that particular antibody which will help their immune system. There was a lot of debate in 2020, on whether they should use it or not because they were concerned about tamping down the immune system if a patient has such a big infection. But their trial data led them to use that drug. It costs about 5,000 thousand per treatment, and they had a discussion about the cost, but found that caring for such patients was already very expensive so that was not an issue. Every day in the ICU would more than cover the cost of this drug. Dr. Kim found it too early to say if the patients are doing well with it. They began using it in early March, but every patient's coronavirus response varies. That is why they meet as a group, and come up with new responses.

Dr. Kim in the Hospital's Operational Structure and the ICU

Dr. Kim is very involved in the hospital's operational structure, and an important member of Incident Command, which occurred during the marathon bombing because they anticipated a large number of people coming into the ICU. It's divided into many branches one of which is the wide operation branch, where a physician is selected to cover all of the ICUs that are usually run separately. Given the demands of the pandemic, they also created a designated survivor of a physician from the ICU. The person in charge of ICU response asked him to keep in touch with him, and promised that there would just be a few meetings per week. However in a few days it grew into a 24/7. He was organizing the ICU care, arranging the physicians' schedules, dealing with supplies, as well as answering clinical guidelines' questions. He worried that they would run out of physicians because there was such a flood of people coming in infected with the coronavirus. There was a special need for someone to sign them into the ICU as well as deciding whether patients were sick enough to come to the critical care unit.

Dr. Kim is very concerned about the variant P.1 in Brazil because it emerged in the city Manaus in early December 2020, and only five weeks later caused a huge surge in cases. Before it arrived in the U.S. it had 75 percent of people infected in Spring of 2020 yet Brazil did not reach herd immunity. While the variant from the U K. took about three months to dominate the outbreak in England, P.1 took only a month in Brazil. One of the scientists who has worked on understanding P.1 found

that that it could infect people who had been vaccinated, and that the
vaccines have to be reformulated or else there is the risk of being
infected twice.[1] Scientists are concerned that P.1 might be more
transmissible and deadlier than the first virus. A public sector research
institute in Brazil found that in 25 of the 27 states more than 80 percent
of intensive care beds were occupied, 18 states had shortages of the
drugs needed to put patients on ventilators, and in six states oxygen
supplies were low. The variant has been discovered in 33 countries.
Although there is insufficient genetic sequencing, studies in Sao Paulo
identified the variant in 80 to 90 percent of cases.[2] President Bolsonaro
downplayed the seriousness of public health measures, and promoted
false cures. As a result the variant has spread widely throughout the Latin
American continent, and now Uruguay, Paraguay, Peru, Argentina and
Colombia are among the top 20 nations in the world with coronavirus
deaths.

A journalist and documentary filmmaker who lives in the Amazon
has written that the Amazon is a global repository of airborne viruses,
and the planet could experience more pandemics. Scientists have
revealed that pathogens are more likely to spread from animal hosts to
humans in deforested areas rather than in healthy bio-diverse forests that
are natural barriers for diseases.[3] President Bolsonaro opened the
Amazon to miners, loggers, cattle ranchers, the construction of highways
and railways. These decisions helped to spread the variant throughout
Brazil.

Dr. Kim found his time in the ICU depressing because patients who
were infected a couple of months ago didn't improve in a few weeks. He
found that if they go into the ARDS phase they can end up on the
ventilator for months, and that while they had new treatments for the
early cases of his patients, they don't have anything else to provide as the
weeks accumulate. He describes what he sees in his patients as *uniquely
horrible*, when it gets to a point that only the ventilator can help them
breathe. That was the time when he knows that they are not going to
recover.

Although Brigham and Women is a hospital that entitled and
privileged people travel to from other states, many of the families in the

ICU are working class immigrants who do not have health insurance or the resources to care for a sick family member at home. He was saddened to tell their patients' loved ones that it was time to let them die. It was the first time that Dr. Kim has seen such a high number of Latino families many of whom needed translators. He was more than touched when family members thanked him for his work. Not many of us realize that people who live in poverty can express their gratitude with such courtesy because they know what suffering is, and don't take anything for granted. Dr. Kim is aware that many people cannot afford health care because he knows about a woman who goes to the emergency room once a month to treat her illness because she has no other choice.

Also because there were so many racial justice issues in 2020, Brigham and Women has done a better job of getting an ethnically diverse population of physicians. They have a few Latino resident physicians, but they need more. They were incredibly helpful during one of the coronavirus surges. For instance, they had a patient who was an undocumented immigrant from Central America. One of the residents was also from that region, and came to the U.S. when he was in high school. When the patient's family needed to have a meeting to inform them that their loved one was dying, he attended it. He was very understanding and talked with them about their similar childhoods, giving them a lot of comfort.

One of the most upsetting things in the early times of the coronavirus was not allowing families to visit their patient. All their communication was by phone or after the patient had died. A frequent and more than difficult reality for Dr. Kim was to see a patient not improving after many weeks, so he and the other physicians prolong the dying. Keeping patients' hearts and lungs on machines while they are getting sicker will not lead to their survival. It's hard for the family to let them die if they weren't there. So they used zoom to have families see how different their loved one looked when they had kidney failure, or when they were proned every few hours to help them breathe, creating lots of pressure wounds such as a big ulcer on the side of their face. They are able to see that their loved one's bodies are there, but not the person they knew. Often nurses are using their own iPhones to communicate with the families. Only in the early months of 2021, did they allow them to see their dying loved one. However, what is still very difficult is that if a patient's family member tested positive, that person could not visit the patient.

The sheer volume of patients has been a challenge. The ICU physicians like Dr. Kim are usually taking care of from 10 to 12 patients, but with the coronavirus patients, they were working with 18 patients at the same time. They may have only a single organ at risk that is like ARDS, and is very familiar to them. The physicians meet with a large group of respiratory therapists and nurses, discussing each patient as they rotate through the ICU rooms. They found coronavirus patients essentially healthy before they became infected. However, many physicians at Brigham and Women are not aware that impoverished patients that may live in the counties of the Rio Grande area in Texas suffer from diabetes and many other co-morbidities, They may have never seen a physician before coming to the ICU.

While they initially focused on the lungs, they were also dealing with unusual problems with one of eight or ten patients having blood clots. The physicians discussed whether they should put a powerful level blood thinner on all of their coronavirus patients as some ICUs did in New York. Some of their patients were given a low-level subcutaneous blood shot which they found safer then giving maximum blood thinners on everyone. One out of 100 patients will have a stroke due to a large blood clot that causes them to die. There are many complications that coronavirus patients deal with besides their lungs. Some of them got secondary infections such as pneumonia. Then there are a whole series of problems patients experience after getting better. One general principle Dr. Kim followed was that if he is intubating patients he would try to use less sedating medicines, because if a patients are intubated for a long time they will be confused from the sedation.

During intubation their patients' lungs relax and they are able to heal. When a patient is extremely ill, their oxygen levels are very low, and paralysis is required to get their muscles extra relaxed. Several times the team would wake up the patient, and lighten the sedation, but often the patient tries to take off the ventilator too soon, and their oxygen levels rapidly decline. Often the team would give patients heavy sedation too deeply for the first couple of months when they are very ill, but then would lighten up the sedation more quickly.

Dr. Kim saw a patient whose arm was swollen and checked him for a blood clot with an ultrasound. It wasn't an obvious clot, but he was worried about it, and they did a test on his hand's circulation. Later that day, a nurse noticed that his left hand wasn't doing well, so a surgeon came in. He was concerned that he may have had an arterial blood clot, that his blood wasn't circulating because of his swollen arm. That night they brought him to the operating room, and left his arm open for a while to watch his control of his hand. Very often they saw a blood clot on an arm or a leg, then put the patient on a maximum dose of blood thinning medications.

Unfortunately, he was so busy that he couldn't comfort some people. He found that when he has a pause, he suddenly has to think about an especially heartbreaking moment. There was a subset of physicians who were not normally working in the ICU that are sharing their thoughts since many of them were depressed or very sad. Because he has been working in pre-coronavirus cases he had experienced so many trying situations. Working as an ICU physician prepared him more because many events took place that are similar to the coronavirus. The emotional moments were when he dealt with families. He had witnessed those times previously in his work at ICU, as a result like other doctors Dr. Kim was able to compartmentalize his days. In his career he learned that if you are not able to a help a patient improve, and then see them become significantly worse, he had to deal with the family, and share what they loved about him or her. When the family left, he had to rush to the next case.

Given Dr. Kim's work in the laboratory, he has been able to have access to scientists who work on genomic sequencing, something that physicians expected the CDC to do, although it allowed them to do their tests locally. He could have accomplished that himself if he wasn't so busy in the ICU and in the Instant Command. Yet in the early days of the pandemic Britain funded a national effort to keep decoding the coronavirus as it spread throughout the country, helping them to trace and end outbreaks, even revealing the origins of the coronavirus. Although the U.S. spends more on biomedical research than any other country, it didn't have the funding.

There was no national effort in the first nine months of the pandemic that could have produced a precise account of how the virus is infiltrating communities through the country. In that time period the U.S. sequenced just 0.4 percent of its coronavirus cases, while the U,K, conducted analysis for 12 percent of its outbreaks. Scientists in the U.S. were dealing with our fragmented health care system, a pandemic response, a lack of coordination, and insufficient federal aid. As the study in Britain revealed, sequencing helps scientists discover not only how the virus is spreading in a particular location, but also how it got there. That is a key source of information essential for curbing the spread of the coronavirus before states, regions and counties become overwhelmed.[4] However, Dr. Kim, and the other physicians were very fortunate to have contact with experts in genomics.

Also they have many sequencing machines, and scientists volunteered doing coronavirus tests for them. Brigham and Women was one of the few hospitals in the country that early in the pandemic could run as many coronavirus tests as they needed. They ran 13 million of them, a unique way of responding to a crisis. Dr. Kim saw that our country and its hospitals needed a huge infrastructure to accomplish regular coronavirus testing. He found them spending all of their time doing what should be a public health job for the country. Also our country is so behind on genomic sequencing because there are insufficient laboratory technicians. Since we do not have enough physicians in our country some of the people who would have done genetic sequencing are working in medical care such as pharmaceutical companies. .

The CDC started doing sequencing at the end of December, but it was a very small amount only a few hundred a week. The numbers rose significantly in March to 9,000 a week, and later President Biden promised to fund 25,000, which is still far lower than Brigham and Women's. It began collaborating with local health laboratories, partnering with the Association of Public Health Laboratories as well as creating contacts with commercial diagnostic laboratories to increase the number of viruses they could sequence. It scaled up its efforts to process specimens from the states every week.[5] However it has a lot of catching up to do since more than 33 million Americans have been infected with the coronavirus.

Throughout the months when Dr. Kim was dealing with so many issues, he wasn't at home, because he was not only working in the ICU, he was working on the operations in the hospital. As a result he had some misunderstandings with his girlfriend who couldn't figure out why he volunteered to work in so many positions. For a couple of weeks in the early days, he decided not to see her in person because he was worried about infecting her while she insisted that it was difficult for her because he had so many responsibilities as a frontline worker. He felt that he couldn't risk seeing people. She lived with family members whose jobs were high-risk, and who were in contact with so many people. For many people seeing their loved ones put his or her job before the people he lived with or cared the most about seemed extreme. She may not have realized that in his busy non-stop schedule many doctors working with coronavirus patients lived separately from their spouses and children for a needed period. He also had some emotional moments with his sister but they came together when he explained his situation with her.

Dr. Kim feels lucky because since he is in contact with physicians and scientists, he doesn't have friends or families who are in denial or unaware of seriousness of the coronavirus. As many physicians and nurses he tries to inform the community where he lives. He has found that generally people agree with science, but won't apply it to their own lives, and think that it is exceptional. For example, he dealt with a patient who was very ill, and who would soon be intubated after he had warned many people not to gather with their family and friends for Thanksgiving, which happened nevertheless. As a result many people tested positive, and were infected with the coronavirus. Then he worked with an older man who went to a bowling ally, and became ill. He found that just bringing in scientific knowledge doesn't work.

We are fortunate to have physicians like Dr. Kim, who has multiple talents that are so important in dealing with the pandemic. He has brought together science and medicine, as well as supporting the hospital's operational structure. With all of his insights, he worked long and demanding hours in the ICU while mentoring newly trained physicians.

A STRANGE LANDSCAPE

Who could have foreseen this strange
landscape; empty apartments
with new locks spelling eviction,
a subway with only a few people,
schools without children, as if a war

had struck without warning, leaving
a new kind of devastation, a tide,
not of refugees, but of a new
and complex disease that is moving
throughout our country like a massive

invasion, that knows no boundaries;
the grandmother who lies dying
in the hospital, the man who cannot
breathe, the young woman who
is unable to walk because the pain

in her muscles turns out to be
caused by blood clots. How do
we navigate this new war zone,
with some people driving a bus
because it is *essential*, some people

working at home, our differences
now magnified, but pain is always
around us like sudden heavy
rain, like wildfires. The soldiers
that are called forth during

this deadly war are doctors, nurses,
emergency technicians who fan
out throughout our country,
like a war zone, yet we are short
of supplies for these soldiers of supplies

for compassion and understanding.

for coming together to face
a pandemic, to move beyond
our differences, arguments, and
denial, to hold each other's hands.

—*Marguerite Guzmán Bouvard*

NURSES

SARAH GHOZAYEL

A Difficult Beginning

Sarah Ghozayel is an emergency room nurse. She started working with Covid-19 patients from the beginning of the outbreak in the Boston area. This was a challenging time when there were so many unknowns about the coronavirus, and healthcare workers had views of the illness that were so different from those of their communities.

In early March; 2020, some hospitals were not prepared with the proper equipment for nurses, and she found that the guidelines about whether a nurse should wear an N95 or a surgical mask kept changing and were based on what was available rather than on their scientific merit. In the early days, nurses wore surgical masks. When N95 masks became available around mid-April, the guidelines changed to wearing them when caring for coronavirus patients. Nurse Ghozayel tried to keep hers as clean as possible, but she saw online that people were using special cover lenses, that come in a paper bag. This didn't really work for her because the inside of the mask was touching what she feared was an infected surface, and she found that the part of the Tupperware bowl she placed over her face worked best.

During the first few months she was very upset to hear people saying that since this pandemic was so unprecedented, medical administrators could not have known what to provide. Because of Boston's reputation for excellent medical care throughout the country she never thought that providing PPEs (personal protective equipment) would be such an issue, and expected that medical personnel would have access to everything that they needed. Surgical masks are not commodities, but now they were hidden and locked away. She felt awful going up to someone requesting permission to get a mask because she needed to protect herself.

In the beginning, it seemed as if Covid-19 was similar to a flu ailment. Nurse Ghozayel was concerned about getting infected, but didn't think that getting it would be the worst- case scenario. She was trying to accept that if she became infected she would be able to manage it since she is young and healthy. However, she was more afraid of spreading it, and her biggest fear is to spread it to her mother-in-law, her mother, or to other patients. Most nurses are afraid of infecting their families.

She found the decision about the lockdown frustrating, having phase one mitigating certain aspects while allowing people to begin going out to many places which gave them a false sense of safety, even though the numbers were trending down. Work remained the same for nurses, and they were still afraid to spread the coronavirus. The outside world was changing, but nurses didn't feel that way. Nurse Ghozayel was still caring for Covid-19 patients, and patients were still testing positive. She found it more than difficult to live between two widely different realities. Her mother relied on the news, and since racism and different political views were taking so much space, she felt that it was over crowding the coronavirus coverage. As a result the coronavirus was rarely written about it during that period, and too few people were concerned about it.

Nurse Gozayel does have conversations about Covid-19, but she finds it a challenge because she doesn't want to upset people. Also she worries about things that people don't even think about. She tries to read the conversation in the room before she says anything. Unfortunately because the coronavirus is such a difficult subject for most people, she tries not to say anything, but it's difficult to escape. She knew that Covid-19 was soaring around the country, but wasn't keeping track as she should have, because while she was concerned about it she was also trying not to think about it at times.

Her brother was in medical school in Florida. She spoke to him almost daily about the differences between Massachusetts and Florida. She finds it really interesting to see how other states are treating the coronavirus. It was only in late June that Governor Ron DeSantis started a program to test staff members in nursing homes and retirement communities. He was even loath to require that people wear masks, and physically distance from each other, quite a difference from Massachusetts in the Spring of 2020.

Her brother was supposed to graduate in August, and her mother was so excited that she wanted everyone to attend. But Sarah Ghozayel argued with her, and told her that she didn't think it was safe to fly in on airplane at the time or even within in a few months. When her mother replied that things were getting better, she told her that nothing had really changed. Fortunately the ceremony was postponed the last week in June. In fact, on July 2, 2020, Florida had single day highs of over 10,000 cases and a forty percent increase of their average the previous week.[1] Many of them were started by close physical contact, and the failure to wear masks during the parties young people attended on the waterfront as well as in their homes. Also the education commissioner issued an order requiring schools to be open full time "for those who require it."[2] This would matter for the homeless and youngsters who live in poverty, but teachers were concerned about being present. To console her mother, nurse Ghozayel showed her how to use FaceTime so she could be with her son.

She graduated with a Masters from Simmons College in the Science of Nursing, but couldn't have her own graduation. She was so looking forward to the ceremony and to celebrating with her friends and family. However, she believes that it is important just to make the best of every situation, and concludes that we live in a technological age where Zoom and FaceTime give us the means to maintain our relationships in this difficult situation.

The Weight of Her Experience

Nurses have a different learning model than physicians. The medical model is diagnosis oriented while nursing is about caring for a patient that requires so much time and attention. Most days she loves being a nurse, but finds that Covid-19 has made her job much more difficult having to constantly change masks and gowns.

She feels fortunate that the chaos that occurred in hospitals in New York during the month of March 2020 did not happen in Boston, and that she faced a lesser mortality rate. She worked briefly in the intensive care unit, and the Covid-19 unit because she was needed there. The ICU in Boston requires a high level of skilled care. There used to be a nurse for every single patient. However that practice was abandoned during the state of emergency, and each nurse worked with a number of patients.

Coronavirus patients are at a high stress level, and nurse Ghozayel knows that it causes even higher stress for the nurses. To help relieve some of that anxiety, the hospital administration recruited people with critical skills and experience. Nurse Ghozayel decided to work a few shifts, and that's where she saw Covid-19 deaths, and people who were on ventilators for weeks and even months with many of them dying. Because nurse Ghozayel faced so many deaths, she didn't sign up for more shifts in order to protect herself.

She is still carrying the burden of that experience. She took care of people that were younger than her mother, and her in-laws, and couldn't help but identify with them. She even felt as if she were one of them, and that it was just a question of circumstance. Nurse Ghozayel didn't tell her family that she was working in the ICU with Covid-19 patients. But when she was arguing with her mother, she told her that there were people younger than her who died, and that she should take this virus more seriously because it was still a big problem.

What nurse Ghozayel learned from her ICU experience is that although she had always worked with nurses, she didn't understand their job until she worked their shifts, and realized the incredible patience required to care for Covid-19 patients. It is not like that in the emergency room where most of the time people are identified and diagnosed quickly, and she could move on. In the ICU, coronavirus patients are so ill and for such a long time that when she would come back a week later she would see the same patients without improvements or sometimes in rapid decline. She found that incredibly frustrating. She wondered how nurses could manage to work in an ICU for long periods of time, and whether they poured their hearts and souls into trying to make their patients feel better or if all they could do for them was to FaceTime their friends and their loved ones. Nobody is allowed to visit them, and spend time with them while they are dying which she found so heartbreaking.

She has cared for a dying patient in the ICU and found that with Covid-19, it is a slow death. When she was in college, she had a course on Death and Dying. It wasn't a class that she had looked forward to, but she was so glad that she did. People need to understand that death and dying is not what a person sees on TV, "a good looking person on a folded sheet that is in bed. It's very ugly." She found that the measures that are taken to keep people alive are almost barbaric, including the use of ventilators, and that these interventions are horribly painful. The ventilators, tubes are inserted in the patient's mouth and forced down into the airway.

She had a lot of conversations with health care proxies, and families about the effects of being on a ventilator for a long period of time. Research has shown that patients suffer from PTSD (Post Traumatic Stress Disorder). They needed help to cope with it as they suffer from long- term effects.

A professor of psychiatry at Columbia University has written about what survival of Covid-19 really means. Patients released from the ICU after extended periods often will have PTSD as well as muscular and neurological problems. To ease the pain of being on ventilators 24/7 for long periods, and to stabilize their breathing patients must be sedated. They cannot move or eat. As a result, their muscles atrophy, and many of them develop kidney injury.[3] Many also suffer from cognitive and mental problems, as well as muscular problems from lying without moving for long periods. Because they are not welcome in nursing homes or long- term rehabilitation centers due to concerns about Covid-19 infections, some of these patients remain in hospitals or return home requiring extensive care.

There was one instance that nurse Ghozayel will never forget. The morning of Mother's Day a woman wasn't getting better, and needed a breathing tube. Since she was the only patient who didn't have a ventilator, there was a little bit of optimism. Unfortunately she declined overnight, and needed to have a breathing tube. They called her daughter, and she held the phone for her, putting her daughter on the speaker. She couldn't help but think that maybe this was the last time that her daughter was going to hear her mother's voice because she might not recover. After that shift, she decided not to work in the ICU. It was too hard so see people dying alone, slowly and painfully.

What nurse Ghozayel has accomplished is to be a caring presence that is so needed by a person who is very ill. She felt that she couldn't accomplish much, but what she did was to offer her care with kindness and concern. Being a very young person striving to do the best she was self-critical.

She now works in two emergency rooms. In the beginning she wanted to be in the ICU but after she applied to both departments, the emergency room called her back first. She felt that her type A personality would be more suited to the ICU, but working in the emergency rooms made her more flexible. She likes it because it is more challenging, and requires very diverse skills. She finds that no two shifts are alike. Sometimes she goes a million miles an hour, sometimes she doesn't, and it can change in a few seconds. Then there are certain procedures and medical care skills that she can use three days in a row, that she may not use them again for another two months, depending on where she is assigned, and which patient she is taking care of. For example, one day she might be caring for a critically ill patient, and the next two hours for a patient who was sexually assaulted. She likes having a broad range of skills.

First she has to determine whether a patient has the coronavirus, and it makes it easier if she already knows that the person has been infected. If she has a patient who was tested positive, a nurse must be safe, to take her time, have her PPE, and decide on an action plan with the physician. The goal is to provide good patient care, but also to maintain her safety that means not having to go into the room ten times an hour. She has to develop a plan with the patient, the doctor, and do her work in an organized and efficient manner. Usually she needs to insert an IV, and do blood work since nurses are good at predicting what blood work they need. Also the staff does vital signs so they can tell if the patient needs an EKG. Sometimes the patients need medications right away, and that is why it is important to coordinate with the physician. Nurses do the nose swabs required to see if the patient is testing positive.

During the first months of caring for Covid-19 patients, the staff was trying to minimize the number of people in the room. In the beginning the nurse was doing everything herself, and some nurses found this exhausting. There were times when they tried to do everything with one nurse, and one provider at their bedside. Caring for a coronavirus patient would be the last place to work because everyone involved might sneeze or cough afterward spreading the aerosols that can infect a person. So it is not wise to be in the room for a long period of time as it increases a nurse's potential exposure.

Nurse Ghozayel is keenly aware of everything that happens around her. For example once she worked with a prisoner in the emergency room. She had been taught that a prisoner's skin integrity is very important. Yet when she pointed out that the handcuffs were too tight on her patient, she was told that keeping the handcuffs on was at the discretion of the accompanying officer, and that they were for her own protection and safety. She was also told that it was not a problem, and although she disagreed she remained silent.

Nurse Ghozayel's ICU shifts lasted 12 hours whereas a nurse works in the emergency room eight to 12 hours usually three or four time a week. She found that wearing an N95 mask for twelve- hour periods was very uncomfortable. In the beginning it was very challenging, but over time she did much better with it, and got fewer headaches. She found that it will always leave marks on your face, but believes that it is important to adapt.

In the beginning nurses were only talking with their co-workers because they were working at the front lines of Covid-19, and felt that they were the only ones that truly understood what was happening. Nurse Ghozayel found that the good that came out of Covid-19 is that physicians, physicians' assistants, and nurses became closer by sharing the same fears and anxieties. She also found it very helpful to support each other informally throughout a person's shift. For her it was humbling, and she enjoyed getting together with people from other disciplines, finding that "it humanized us." Everyone came together as a team, sharing the attitude that they were all in this together and would support each other.

Nurse Ghozayel learned other things that were not appealing, such as how much our health care system responds to money. She noticed that professional athletes were able to get quick access to testing, and wondered why only the rich and famous get quickly tested, but others don't. Actually, in many states there are lines that stretch for miles with people waiting to be tested. It seems absurd to her that as an asymptomatic person she cannot get a test despite that fact that she is taking care of people who are Covid-19 positive. Like many health workers she worries about being at risk.

Nurse Ghozayel also had questions about whether hospitals really care about its nurses. She feels that their priorities were not right when the administrators seem to be more focused on the aesthetics of the hospital by putting flower arrangements in the halls rather than providing sufficient PPEs for the medical personnel. Actually, most hospitals are run for profit, and their executives receive very high salaries. The medical staff where she worked received many food donations and other gifts from businesses that helped so much to boost their morale. Some stores even offered discounts to health care workers. She remarked that "it feels like a stranger cares about you more than your work place does."

The hospitals where she works offered supportive meetings on Zoom. There was a nightly check in, around eight o'clock in the evening when anyone from any discipline could check in on the meeting. It was a way of releasing the overwhelming emotions that arise from caring for Covid-19 patients. She found that both of the hospitals where she worked really did try to address the mental health issue. There are so many differences in the care that hospitals offer nurses and patients.

However, given the fact that there was no consistent leadership from the previous administrations regarding testing, contact tracing, social distancing and mask wearing some states have opened up too soon, and found themselves in sudden need for a quick responses to the surge of the virus in July, 2020. Unlike countries in Europe, there is no social safety net for the millions of unemployed. The House and Senate did pass a relief measure to help the unemployed and small businesses, but it expired at the end of July, although in Massachusetts it was extended until the end of October 2020. Also with the new administration in 2021, health care workers are being supported in many ways.

In states that have seen high numbers of new cases such as Florida, Arizona, California and Texas, hospitals are finding themselves overwhelmed in a number of ways. For example, Florida has rushed 100 new health-care workers to Miami Dade's public hospital including 75 nurses to work in ICU.[4] As well as dealing with staff and space in the hospitals there has been a shortage of protective gear, emergency room waits have grown, and ICUs are filled or almost near capacity. Given the surge, nurses often extend their twelve- hour shifts without being told to do so. Some hospitals are also reshuffling their staff and some are implementing "just in time" training to boost their staff.[5] This is something that upsets nurse Ghozayel so much that she would rather not talk or even think about it because she is so concerned about her patients.

Nurse Ghozayel did talk to her husband, and her mother about it although a lot less months later because it became part of her life, and was unfortunately the new normal.

Nurse Ghozayel is only twenty-seven. She has been a nurse for five years. Although she is still very young, she has acquired a lot of strength and hope. She has learned something that only people who have experienced in difficult times that a person can live with both sadness and contentment.

TAMATA KABA

Going Into the Trenches

Tamata Kaba is a neuroscience nurse at the Brigham and Women's hospital in Massachusetts. When the coronavirus appeared she was working on the neuroscience unit in the intermediate floor, and then moved to the ICU unit in March 2020 to take care of patients with a new and overwhelming illness. At that time they were receiving emails that the coronavirus was spreading, but they did not know what it was. Thus the hospital was trying to inform other places about the nature of this new illness. New York City hospitals were calling for nurses because they were desperately in need of help, so she left her staff position, and ended up going to Queens New York as a travel nurse in the ICU, and worked there until May.

She found it very frightening going to New York as a travel nurse. She told her family, and they were very upset, but something in her heart was saying "just do it." She remembers being in her house, putting all of her things in the car, and then taking the four-hour drive from Massachusetts to New York. She was nervous, but also praying because she is a person of deep faith. She was afraid of being on a coronavirus floor. Unfortunately at this time there were insufficient PPEs, but she insisted that she would not go there without PPEs and N95s that were in great demand.

When she arrived at the hospital she was given more than she asked for; a hair bonnet, a face shield, an N95, and a surgical mask. She also was provided with a double gown, with one in front and one in back, double gloves with one pair going up our arms so that nothing was able to be in contact with her skin. She even had feet coverings. Previously, nurses were supposed to bring in their own uniforms. Luckily, they were having many donations at that time so ICU nurses were properly covered.

Despite the danger, nurse Kaba found it was such a pleasure to be there because there were so many people working together. But when she took the subway to the hospital she was very nervous. As soon as she arrived, she went to her unit to get her assignment, and then off to her designated work place. They dedicated the whole top floor of the hospital to the nurses. Also at this time few people seemed to know what the virus was, and as a result a lot of bed and breakfasts were afraid of their homes being contaminated so it was not easy to find a place to stay for the travel nurses. Everything was in a state of change because of the fear and uncertainty about the coronavirus.

Given the fact that there was no leadership from the federal government in the previous administration, cases proliferated in January and February. There was no testing, and contact tracing that was needed throughout the country not only in New York. Also Governor Andrew Cuomo and Mayor Bill de Blasio did not close the schools, restaurants and other services in time. Researchers found that thousands of lives could have been saved in the city if these policies had been taken just a week earlier.[1]

When nurse Tamata Kaba came to New York City, she found a very different landscape because there were so many closures, and the city was on lockdown that made it seem like a dessert. There were no cars, no people, and even homeless people were out of sight. When she walked out of her hotel into Times Square which used to be one of the most populated streets, it was empty except for army personnel trying to make sure that there was order, and that people were wearing masks. It was a dreary sight. Then when she took the subway wearing her uniform to get to work, people would look at her a little strangely as if she had the virus.

But the camaraderie from the fire department for all of the travel nurses, the doctors, the travel nurse practitioners, and the lobotomists was very uplifting. Also, when they would go into their shifts, people would stand outside of their apartment buildings, sing and clap for them, banging on their pots and pans as a way of cheering and thanking them. It was a wonderful experience, and there were signs thanking them in so many places. If they would see her, they would come up, and say "thank you for your service." She found it heart wrenching because that is what we say to the veterans when they come home from war. Nurse Tamata Kaba felt that people saw nurses as if they were heroines because they were working in the trenches. She felt that she was just putting her arms around the patients, saying that she was going to help them.

Even just trying to get out of her hotel room for a walk was troubling, and she found that strolling in Times Square was walking in a depressing landscape. Besides that all the stores were closed. She went into a Thai restaurant, and saw the owner tying up all her receipts, looking worried. She wondered about some of the restaurants that were open despite the fact that we are in the middle of an apocalypse, and whether she could trust that her takeout was clean. But she also saw that small businesses were closed at the time, and knew that they must have invested so much money, and the few that were open were probably in danger of closing. Yet people were still donating food, and all of the small restaurants were feeding them, even though they were losing their business.

The first day she entered the hospital, there were nurses everywhere and she didn't even have an orientation at this point. Yet as a travel nurse you have to know how to handle whatever awaits you, so she is comfortable wherever she goes, even outside of the U.S. she is fine working with a critically ill person. "You walk into a war zone, put on your PPE, where they had a lot of doctors and nurses, and you knew that this was a strictly Covid-19 unit. Then you put on your gear, and walk into this unit, thinking, God, you are with me."

The first time she walked into the ICU there were nurses everywhere amid a great deal of chaos. In fact every day was chaotic, but she is a very calm person, and nothing jolts her. She is used to seeing death all of the time. But the numbers kept increasing so fast that it was difficult to deal with, plus there were so many ICU patients.

Typically in an ICU there is a one nurse to one patient ratio, which is a lot of work, and if they are dying you are with them every second. Now she was getting three patients, and some nurses had three or four sick patients. Yet she knew that such a traumatic environment was not going to overtake her. There were many nurses taking that horrible scene home with them. She never did that because even though she was part of a team that cares for them. Because the coronavirus is so unpredictable, she knew that she couldn't go home with those feelings like so many nurses. Many of them would go home, and think about how they could have done more. She saw a lot of depression, and a lot of people feeling overwhelmed with so many patients needing so much care. But she also saw the bigger picture, that she was there to help, and that she did her best. Yet she was concerned about the toll it took on her co-workers. If that is what a nurse sees day after day it will hurt her in many ways if she can't handle it. She wondered if there would be counseling for them because patients were dying at such a high rate. She also wondered what services hospitals were going to provide for the nurses, because seeing that everyday is a grave challenge.

Nevertheless, she found it an amazing environment to work in because it was so unpredictable, and so difficult that all of the nurses were so appreciative of travel nurses. They thanked them for their help because they were so swamped. The surgical floor was turned into an ICU, forcing nurses to learn new skills amidst the chaos. Coming from the Brigham and Women's' hospital taught her how to be a rock in such a challenging situation. She would walk in the room she was assigned to, and ask who would be in charge. Then she was told that she would be the one who would run things to make sure that everything goes smoothly, and to find the patients who were the most critically ill.

When the doctors came in at midnight to do their rounds and decide which patient would get intubated, and in the morning when they arrive to see the conditions of the critically ill patients, the charge nurse would come in. It meant a lot because they trusted her to be in that role even though they had never met her. The floor they had never used before was set aside for the ICU was like a wide-open gymnasium. Every bed was occupied and every inch of that gymnasium was filled with nurses, and patients that were intubated and sedated. Yet nurse Tamata Kaba wanted to be in the trenches. She was grateful, and made wonderful friends because they were all nervous, and didn't know much about the coronavirus. Everyday they would hug each other. Nursing in such a situation taught her that life is so short and unpredictable.

They dedicated the whole top floor of the hospital to nurses. There was a lot of fear in the hospital. Patients would come in with breathing problems. She remembers a man that came in who was in his early forties, telling her that he was having a little shortness of breath, and she was assigned to him. At the beginning of her shift she was giving him oxygen because his oxygen was low, but he seemed fine, and was even talking to her.

His wife called in at the front desk and nurse Kaba told her that his oxygen saturations were a little low, but that he was doing all right. She responded by asking her to give her husband her love. Nurse Kaba's shifts are from seven pm. to seven am. She found that the man went down pretty quickly, from the normal 90 percent to 88 percent. Around midnight she paged the doctor to come to his bedside He started by giving him nasal cannula, then high flow oxygen because it is one level higher, behind his back well as in his nose. She remained by his bedside, getting all the medications that he needed, the scapula and the endotrachial tube to go into his throat so he could get intubated. She was stunned by his rapid decline. Previously she had held the hands of people that were losing their loved ones in her work, because as a neuroscience nurse, people died of strokes or brain injuries.

She worked on both the Step Down Unit and the ICU. At the Step Down Unit they gave the patient high flow to get oxygenated. When they declined and needed more help they were sent to the ICU and placed on the ventilator. Then she gave them their medications, took their blood pressure, and gave hourly output checks. Usually, in an ICU, she would document every hour, the input and the out take, urination, and vomiting. She would do urological checks on her patients, or decrease the sedation to see if they could be woken up. During the pandemic it was not done because the patients were in such critical condition. The doctors and department managers told the nurses to document once, and just keep the patients alive. There was no way a nurse could document hourly given the five or six patients under her care. It was a necessary adjustment.

At that hospital the nurses had more autonomy, and she was performing more tasks than she was used to. As an ICU nurse she is able to work in different parts of the hospital, but in the ICU the patients needed more attention when they were intubated. There were new ones that she hadn't seen before because there was a shortage of nurses, and needed to be shipped from different places. It was new territory for the machines that they used, as well as the care that the patients were getting.

Nurse Kaba was also proning and bathing the patients, waiting at their bedside for the physicians if they needed more medication.

When patients were intubated she would see that her patients had a lot of emphysema which is a build up of fluid in their lungs, which could be pneumonia. She would then give them CPR (cardiologic pulmonary resuscitation) pushing down on the patients' chests, then when she lifted her finger, she found that the imprint for her fingers would still be there because there was so much fluid. She found that if she lightly massaged, she could feel the air crackle like emphysema that has so much fluid in the lung cavity, something she had never seen before. They had the patients supine with the head of their bed slightly raised, so that their lungs could drain. But they found that the fluid in their bodies couldn't be released, and was just going into different cavities so parts of their bodies were swollen. They also had blisters in different places under the bed linen as a result.

If they weren't responding to that with their ultra saturation, and if the patients who were intubated were not where they wanted them to be, they would start proning them, which includes putting their patients on their bellies to give their lungs in back some time to adjust. She found proning very difficult because if her patient was lying on his face or on his back there could be skin breakdown, and she worried about that. The nurses would put cushions around their foreheads, chins, elbows and kneecaps to help the places around the bones. She saw so many patients in that condition.

Nurse Tamata Kaba would do a lot if CPR when a patient's heart stops beating, and she checked the pulse and the cardiac artery on both sides of the neck. If someone stops breathing, and their heart stops pumping, the nurses pump all of the left side of the chest close to the heart on the left side to keep the heart working until it fills the whole body with oxygenated blood. When that happens, all of the vital organs aren't getting any oxygen or blood. Patients also get ventricular tic, a heart that is beating so fast, they also have to do a CPR. Doing a CPR creates an air flow through the diaphragm and rib cage, and often the doctors wouldn't risk that because they didn't want to get infected.

The ICUs were newly established so nurse Tamata Kaba would scan her floor when she started her shift to see where all the supplies were; the blood draws, the needles, the Codes in case her patient had one, and the telemetry machine to check her patient's heart and blood pressure. She found that every day was unpredictable and she would need different supplies. If a patient was dying, they created the last scene with so much care. She remembers a 94-year old woman who was from the Philippines, and couldn't speak English which was typical of the demographics where patients spoke Spanish or Creole. She spent a lot of her time staying next to patients who had difficulty breathing which she found frightening, a setting that broke her heart. She stayed by a patient, holding her hand, and talking to her quietly trying to give her hopeful words even if she thought she couldn't understand English. For the patients, the sound of caring voice can be soothing even when she or he is dying. She treated every patient as a member of her family, finding it heart wrenching.

She also spoke to a lot of family members who would call for updates, and gave them a lot of moral support, telling them that she understood. Family members were thanking her for taking care of their loved ones all the time. Often they were crying, and she would cry with them. She was talking to a least three family members one after the other throughout the whole night. They all wanted to hear that their family member who was intubated was alive, and that they still had a heart beat.

Reflections On Her Time in New York

When nurse Tamata Kaba left New York, she asked herself what her purpose was, and found that she is on this earth to tell people that they have one life to live, and they have to live it to the fullest. Although she is only thirty years old, she has always thought of deeper things. Despite the fact that her time this did not take an emotional toll on her, mentally she felt that she had grown, and that she needed to go to New York. She didn't want to continue her work in Massachusetts, but rather to have new horizons and travel. She prays, and meditates. Her inner world is at peace despite having been in such a trying place.

She was there for eight weeks. After that she thought that life is too short, and even when she wants to complain about things, she reflects on how fortunate she is that she has two arms, two legs, and can still breathe on her own. She has learned to be appreciative of life and to be mindful. She found that living with death and suffering day after day is a learning experience, and that there is more than being frightened and experiencing sorrow. It took a toll on people working there, but she is so grateful that she was there and able to help out. She learned how precious life is.

Tamata Kaba is West African and Lebanese. Her mother is from Sierra Leone, is part Lebanese, and was raised in Free Town, Sierra Leone while her grandmother raised five children alone. Her father is from Guinea. She was born in the U.S., and is proud of her heritage and her family, despite living with bigotry. She is very independent and dedicated to learning and serving people in need. She rose above the prejudices she faces concluding that everyone should respect each other, and understand our differences. She believes in living with love, honesty and integrity that she has always had to be strong. She knew that she would be a dedicated person who calls herself a warrior. Growing up with the Muslim faith, she understands the difference between racism and culture, knowing that children don't grow up racist, but that it was taught to them.

Tamata Kaba studied at Massasoit Community College, but wanted to continue her studies, and applied to the University of Massachusetts in Boston. The Chairman of Neuroscience at the Massachusetts General Hospital headed a scholarship program, Collaborative of Leadership Nursing that was given to minority nursing students in order to help diversify the Partners Healthcare System. She was fortunate to be one of the four applicants who received one. She graduated in 2016, and began her first job as a neuroscience nurse at the Newton Wellesley Hospital.

She is grateful for having had that experience in New York City. She is proud of being African, and is deeply faithful. Her grandmother had an important influence on her since she is a Muslim, yet also attended Christian Churches. Tamata Kaba blends her Muslim faith with Buddhism. She believes in what she refers to as abundance, giving what one has to others.

SHIRLEY BRUCELAS

Grief and Strength Intertwined

From the moment nurse Shirley Brucelas was transferred from her original department in OBGYN to a section for patients with the coronavirus, she worked with great strength and compassion, despite the outpouring of emotions she experienced in such a setting. Usually, it is Pastors, Rabbis, Imams, and psychiatrists who work with people facing death. But for a nurse to be suddenly placed in such a dire situation she must comfort and console her patients as well as dealing with all of the emotions she is experiencing for the first time. Since families of the patients are not allowed to be with them, this can be a harrowing task. Grief and strength are intertwined, and Nurse Brucelas has accomplished this by letting her feelings pour out, then returning to her work that she regards as so important.

When she was deployed in early March 2020, she was not at all prepared since she had never worked in an ICU before. At a time when the coronavirus infected so many people in New York and the hospitals were overwhelmed, there was insufficient staff to respond, so they were hired from clinics. Nurse Brucelas found herself with cascading emotions such as fear and uncertainty, not knowing what to expect. But she reminded herself that she was in the medical field, and that she chose to be a nurse, "but when it comes to something as serious as the Covid-19, she reflected, you can't help but think about your own safety, and that of your family." In fact, her husband had lost his sense of smell and taste, but had tested negative, happening at a time when testing wasn't being done. As a result she isolated herself for 14 days.

She was concerned about the availability of masks because she read newspaper articles about the lack of masks and the PPE equipment (protective personal equipment). But she was assured by her superior that she would have it. In fact the minute she walked in, they took her temperature, and gave her a brown bag with an N95 mask. Once she arrived at her unit she received the remaining PPE equipment, the face shields, gowns, and gloves.

It was very challenging to enter a Covid-19 ward. She had so many questions, but then told herself, "This is what it is. Take it or leave it." She found the new job really frightening and compared her first shift to a roller coaster ride. In her words, "You go in and you set your mind, I am going to do this without knowing what the outcome will be, and how you will feel the moment in time when you get on this ride."

Nurse Bruchelas was placed on a 12-hour night shift three days a week. She found it to be a difficult adjustment. Not only were the hours and shifts challenging, but her emotions were often overwhelming, including grief and anger. She was her own source of support, and achieved it by talking to herself, saying that it was something that she had to do, that she would face it and work hard. But she also had concerns about how she could protect herself. But again she was the one to respond to her worries, "I can't help others if I am not well myself," and continually reminded herself that could handle this demanding job.

The first assignment they gave her was on the Covid-9 floor. She remembers walking in where everyone was wearing PPEs from head to toe, all the patients rooms were filled with contact precautions, and signs on the closed doors. It was overwhelming. At ten o'clock, she broke down, and told the staff that she needed a minute because the rapid response calls she would hear overhead were going on continually. She knew that a rapid response was not a good outcome, and meant that a patient was dying. She found it very frightening.

The first night on her shift she cried, and told the staff she needed a few minutes. She was overwhelmed, and took all the PPE off, which in itself was difficult because it made her hot and sweaty. She found that trying to breathe properly through all of this equipment while trying to take care of struggling patients was not an easy task. To deal with that she talked to herself about acceptance, and how to protect her family as much as possible when she came home.

One of the most difficult parts of her job was to accompany the dying, keeping them company, and making them as comfortable as possible during their last moments. It was not an easy task. Sometimes her emotions soared right in the middle of her work. That first night shift was like a war zone. It felt surreal. It was a battle with a disease that was taking lives in such a rapid manner. Friends of hers died that were healthy, and although she heard that it was people of a certain age who were at risk of dying, she found that it happens to all ages. She also heard stories of staff members who came down with the illness and died. In addition, she felt that she had PTSD (post traumatic stress disorder) because she became very cautious, about what she touched, constantly washing her hands, not touching her face, being very aware of the dangers of contagion. She had to tell this to her patients, to let them know how to protect themselves. She told them that gloves were not protecting them. When they leave, they touch their cars, doorknobs, and phones. If they kept wearing their gloves, they were not protecting themselves, but making it worse. She knew that she when she returned to her house she needed to sanitize her car and phone. At the time she felt that the news was not providing enough information about how to protect themselves, especially those who have had contact with persons who were infected with the coronavirus.

Nurse Brucelas discovered that in a world where everyone is vulnerable seems like a war zone. She taught herself new things every day. However, it is very difficult to return from a war zone. For example when a veteran of the war in Iraq, saw a tin can in the road where she was driving in her home town, she was terrified because she thought it was an IED (improvised explosive device).

Everyday was a new experience for Nurse Brucelas while she learned and adjusted, and every shift was different. She could not predict what was going to happen, and learned that she had to be prepared for anything and everything. Once again, she constantly told herself, that as long as she had her PPE, and removed it accordingly, she was doing her best to stay as Covid-19 negative as possible in order for her to get through the night and her shift. She developed a process to disinfect herself once she returned to her home. When she arrived at the entrance of her front door, she put her uniform in a bag and put Lysol everywhere because she was concerned about her children who lived with her and her husband.

She thinks that she did a good job taking care of her patients. She discovered that all these dangers didn't matter because she had so many patients who were so afraid. Young men who were in their forties were so concerned when she was going through their vital signs that they needed to be reassured. She would tell them that they were in a hospital environment, were in good hands, and would make it through. She had some patients who tested positive, and became so depressed because they couldn't leave the hospital since they had no place to stay. Some of them were homeless and lived in shelters so they needed more services.

She learned that being infected also brings up so many mental issues. She helped a woman whose oxygen level was not good, but became so conscientious that she would hyperventilate because she was so uncomfortable with the oxygen off. After 14 days of being there she told Nurse Brucelas, "I've come a long way," but now she told her that she needed oxygen because she was so afraid of facing death. It was a challenge every night, and she had to prepare herself to say. "I know you're afraid, but you just have to do the best you can and keep going."

Since there were no visitors allowed, patients were dying alone. She would help other nurses who were attending dying patients, preparing and wrapping the body, a process which she found devastating. She remembers a time when the Codes were so frequent that the nurses felt more than drained. The constant repetition of rapid response Codes were overwhelming, but it became the norm. Code is a rapid response when a patient is deteriorating, either not breathing properly, or going into cardiac arrest. That is when doctors and nurses with advanced training respond to a severe emergency situation. The nurses on the floor will start the CPR (Cardio Pulmonary Resuscitation) until the rapid response team arrives. When that happens, every second counts, and people have to move quickly. They start with putting a board behind the patient's back to give them support while giving chest compression. A patient won't get a good compression if they are laying down. The team gives them heart medication, heavy fluids, and emergency resuscitation, trying to do the best they can to revive the patient.

While Nurse Brucelas was in the Covid-19 ward, so many patients were dying that there was a constant rapid response. At the end of April it became so overwhelming and depressing that they implemented a happy quote. Whenever anyone would either leave the hospital as Covid-

19 positive, or would be taken off of the ventilator, they would announce the happy quote. It was wonderful to hear about some patients recovering or going home in the midst of so many people dying.

Nurse Brucelas also worked in the emergency room where a patient would be screened for any signs or symptoms of the virus. The nurses would automatically do the swabbing of the nose, to find out if they tested positive for the virus regardless of whether they had the symptoms. What she found alarming was that people were still testing positive even if they didn't have any symptoms. As a result they had to treat everyone who came into the emergency room as a risk. They would do a rapid review of the test so it would become a stat with the word stat on a red bag, meaning that it should be done immediately. The results would come in a couple of hours, and placed on the patient's chart. The nurses would try to keep them isolated. She found that March was chaotic, and that Covid-19 was widespread in the emergency room.

In April when things slowed down a bit the nurses tried to confine Covid-19 positive patients to a certain area of the emergency room. They needed to keep them more confined to avoid the spread. The amount of people coming in with these symptoms, and dying was overly high. For example, a person would come in with breathing issues who was not in good shape, and died. For most of the patients it was too late, as they were dying of complications of the virus in the emergency room. At the end of the week there was a very high number of deaths, something that is unusual there.

One of the terrible discoveries was that the morgue section of the hospital wasn't able to hold the bodies. Nurse Brucelas was surprised at the small size of that area. As a result they had to get help from the outside, relying on ice trucks to take them. She found it inhumane to put the bodies in a bag, only to deposit them in the truck. She heard from her coworkers that a worker from a funeral home came to pick up a body with bags. This was, a new practice that was certainly not a normal procedure for a family or a funeral home. Unfortunately it was a response to the number of people coming into the emergency room. They didn't have time for the proper protocol in just a half hour.

No families were allowed in the emergency room when Covid-19 started. It was very painful for them because staff member were telling them that their family member was not doing very well. Then a doctor would come outside, informing them that they had lost their loved one, a very difficult message at a time when the details of the coronavirus was not widely known. Nurse Brucelas was distressed that the health care system not well prepared for such an outbreak. She regards the whole process as more viable now, but believes that it needs to be revamped, and create a more viable plan.

There was one shift in the ICU that Nurse Brucelas felt was the worst shift she ever participated in. She was alone with six other nurses taking care of patients who were on ventilators, and thus needed full time care. They had to turn patients over every two hours to help them breathe, and also to wash them, because some of them were in a coma. Some of were not doing very well, and were in bad shape. She remembers one patient that was in the early stages of dying, and that his blood sugar was very low. They were giving him medications to raise it, but it wasn't working. As a result the doctor called the family warning them that there were more complications, and that the patient might not survive. The family's children were very upset because they may not have realized that their loved one had such a life threatening illness.

It was very demanding for a nurse to communicate with family members because they could misinterpret certain words. Also they may have thought that their loved one was doing well, and were surprised by the phone call. To receive a call in the middle of the night, or in the early hours of the morning seems unusual at a time when the danger of being ill with the coronavirus was still so new. This can be frustrating for both the doctor and the family since it's difficult to face death when its unexpected, and happening in such a short period of time. There was not that much information available to the public in March. Plus during the early months of the coronavirus physicians weren't sure if they could admit family members in the early stages of dying.

Although at the time, there was a widespread belief that older people were the most at risk for becoming infected, she found that there were all ages in the ICU, including a 21 year old woman who died, a few in the mid-thirties, as well as the elderly. There was also a mixture of races, Hispanic, African American and Caucasian. She found it an eye-opener. It made her worry about her own health since so many minorities do not have the option of living in good health with medical insurance and decent housing. Nurse Brucelas knows that such a life style is very expensive, and finds it very sad.

To ensure that she would remain in good health she spent a lot of time making her home clean even when she is getting ready for work. It became an added stress. She would come in to the hospital, wearing a glove just to open the main door. And she developed a routine such as having her temperature taken before heading to the nurse's station for her assignment. Then, she would take off her gloves, clean her hands, punch in, put on another pair of gloves and press the button for the elevator. She even used wipes for the floor plus making sure she would clean the computer she used around the ward, completely sanitizing it, including the keyboard. She would even do that to the sanitizer that was on the wall, and kept looking at the other nurses hands. She now understands that these precautions are a part of PTSD.

Nurse Brucelas has two children, aged 22 and 18 whom she still calls "her babies." She wanted to be able to hug her daughter and express her love. That change was something very difficult to give up. Not many people think of how our doctors and nurses need to keep a distance from their families when returning from the hospital, and how painful it is. Loving families are a source of support.

Coming Back From War

Although Nurse Brucelas no longer works with Covid-19 patients, she still behaves in the same way, even at home and with her car. She took a train to the city which seemed like progress. A veteran from our recent wars uses similar signs as progress. Too many nurses in the in the emergency room died when she was in the early period of treating coronavirus patients. Many people believe that PTSD wears off, but it can last for years.

She remembers that one of the nurses was insufficiently prepared. At that time, they did not have access to protective equipment such as N95s. Regular surgical masks were not protective for such a severe illness. In

March it started affecting so many people in New York City. She saw a photo of a Philippine nurse in every ward, who had worked in the emergency room and died of Covid-19. Her coworkers explained that the nurse was already feeling sick, and had contacted a doctor she worked with. He didn't want to test her so she called her primary care doctor. He told her to go home and quarantine. In less than a week she died. There was insufficient manpower at the time so if a patient could breathe on her or his own, and wasn't dying, they were just told them to go home. Nurse Brucelas found that they were treating it as if it were a cold, telling them to keep hydrated, and to come back if they still had shortness of breath. She felt that too many people died that could have been saved.

There was a shortage at that time, and the staff needed to take equipment from the clinics, closing some of them, taking their PPEs where she was in OBGYN. She saw a nurse wearing an N95 for an entire week, though it is only safe for one use.

Nurse Brucelas received her PPE in the beginning of April. The Covid-19 infections had already started in January, and she felt that there were too many months when the staff didn't protect nurses and patients. When she was sent to work in the emergency room she had told her supervisor if she didn't receive sufficient PPEs, she would leave her job.

This was a time when testing was insufficient, and when the former president told the governors that they needed to increase their efforts to secure medical supplies. For example, Governor Hogan who was a Republican, and his wife who was from South Korea, negotiated with suppliers in that country to obtain testing kits. They received a large number so that they could not only help their health workers, but also test patients in nursing and group homes. In addition that helped them create expanded drive-through sites, primary care practices, and urgent care centers. Other states that were desperate for PPEs and other medical supplies quietly moved to acquire it from other countries.[1]

It was only in July 2020 that the administration proposed a new strategy for testing since there were cars lined up for miles with people waiting. The new type of testing, pooled testing, was decades old, but would reach more people and would be available by the end of the summer of 2020. The United States used this technique around the world at its military bases. What inspired this decision was the alarming rise of cases. Pooled testing was used in China, Germany, Israel and Thailand with more than 2.5 million tested in Beijing due to a new outbreak.[2] A few states such as Nebraska had already started this. It could be used in universities, schools seeking to open, and religious organizations, places where infections were expected be low. Physicians disagreed on the usefulness of such testing because it is not diagnostic, yet many states were open to this kind of testing. What makes this so difficult is that the overall response to the pandemic was polarized between some states, and the administration.

Nurse Brucelas feels that she learned a lot and feels positive. Helping patients was very comforting for her, especially when she saw them recover, and heard their stories about how long they were in the hospital. Seeing them get better was very rewarding.

Working with Covid-19 was a shock because it was not something a medical person was prepared for. She has not talked about her experience to anyone. Now that she is back in her department, the manager asked her how it was and she responded, "horrible." The manager assured her that they were trying to develop a place, and personnel where she could have someone to talk to. Everyone around a person who works with coronavirus patients are worried about them, especially after learning that she cannot hug or kiss her children or that sometimes she had to stay in isolation for a while because she didn't want to infect her husband. In order to protect them she didn't want them to hear about so many deaths.

Although she stopped working with Covid-19 patients, she still behaves in the same way, at work, at home and with her car. Even being in a supermarket was a move upward, and taking a train to go into the city for the first time was very important for her. She took a picture of it for her daughter while she texted her. She is taking small steps to get back into ordinary life, but is still washing everything. A soldier from our recent wars uses similar signs as progress

Like a veteran returning from the battlefield, it is not always possible to translate that experience to those of our daily lives where death and suffering does not intrude in such high numbers. It is difficult for a nurse like Shirley Brucelas to process all that has happened where a month or a trying week will carry the weight of decades. There is both the desire to protect loved ones, and the new ways of behaving that are different from their previous lives. It will take time to visit a zoo, to admire the play of light on a sidewalk near a tree, or to walk in the park. They should be decorated and honored like our veterans who carry the emotional and mental scars of war.

Before this time of working with Covid-19 patients, Nurse Brucelas found that nursing was not highly regarded, but the work coronavirus patients has made nurses heroines and heroes because they put their lives on the line. Everyone who is involved are putting themselves in harms way, something that needs to be respected, honored, and understood.

Many nurses like Shirley Brucelas and New York emergency room technicians felt the devastating signs of mental health problems. In fact the World Health Organization issued a report about the coronavirus' impact on the vulnerability of health care workers to depression, insomnia, and anxiety. These problems don't ago away and last for a long time. As the need for such intensive care grows, so does the adrenaline that keeps them working under such difficult conditions. It took some time before hospitals began to provide psychological care for the medical personnel, so nurses like Shirley Brucelas had to move back to normality on their own.

Unfortunately, too many people are unaware of the emotional and psychological burden of caring for patients who are dying alone, and for the tremendous efforts nurses have made to help them, such as singing to them, holding their hands, accompanying them with great tenderness when they die without the presence of their families. Then they have to quickly move on to the next patient, and are unable to take a solitary break just to cry. Many nurses who no longer work with coronavirus patients refuse to talk about their experiences because they are too painful, just like many soldiers who remain silent about the horrors that they experienced in a war zone. Our medical personnel are like our soldiers who have returned stateside from Afghanistan and Iraq, who suffer from PTSD, with many who commit suicide, and yet our society is unaware of their trauma.

BRENDA HALLOUM

A Challenging Career

Brenda Halloum is an ICU nurse who works in a Texas hospital on a 12 hour shift. During the months of late June and July 2020 when the hospital was overrun with Covid-19 patients she worked 16 hours and sometimes more. But she was not provided with the equipment she needed to protect herself from infection, and had to order reusable N95 masks because at that time the hospital was not providing the PPEs (personal protective coverage) and she would have to use her regular gown. Also she would get just a tubing twist and IV lines to use outside of the room that didn't have negative pressure required for the treatment of coronavirus patients. Unfortunately they didn't have doors on 14 of the 20 ICU rooms. If the nurses did have to go into the rooms at the time, they would take off their gowns, masks and wipe all of their equipment after they left, but there were times when they couldn't, and had to rush to the next patient. Also when she stayed in that room for post mortem care, she came out drenched after doing chest compressions. She used the same mask three days in a row and sometimes for three weeks until her reusable N95 arrived. She bought it with her own money.

Many times when she came out of those rooms she thought that she had gotten infected. Her husband who is a pulmonologist was also exposed every time that he went to work. They were both worried about getting tests, and not wasting them. She was tested just twice. If she came home he would just assume that he would also be tested negative. In February, 2020 he was one of the first to wear N95 masks. People would stare at him, wondering why he was wearing them, and he told Brenda that there were hospitals that didn't have masks or gloves.

There is a day care at the hospital where she works in Brownsville, Texas, but she has a family friend that helps her for three days a week. She has five children, two-year old twins, a seven year old, an eleven year old and a twelve year old. When she comes home from the hospital she leaves everything in the garage, strips down, and takes a shower. The children all know not to come in contact with her, and that her area in the garage is off limits. Nor were they allowed to touch her shield that she bought as well as the protective goggles. She also ordered some shields for the department when they were limited with just masks.

On her days off, she would do research about her new equipment. According to what she read, they were supposed to dry clean their reusable masks in order to reuse them. Since she didn't think that was sanitary, she would look up face shields and goggles, then bought a collection that she tried. She did a lot of research for the proper protective gear.

In fact Bonnie Costillo, the head of National Nurses United is very active both in securing equipment for nurses that didn't receive it, but also working on behalf of nurses, giving talks on the lack of equipment. She is also active in providing masks not only for nurses but also for people like teachers who are in dire need of them. She is continually on twitter and other social media on behalf of the nurses. But nurses like Brenda Halloum did not have time for this because she was overwhelmed with work, and didn't receive the medications that would help her patients or enough information about the coronavirus.

When the pandemic broke out there was a national shortage of masks, PPEs, gloves, and face shields so that nurses were dying As a result they started protesting around the country, and held evening candle light vigils for the nurses who died as well as demanding life saving equipment. Also there was a lot of fake equipment that was sold. The FBI related that this was an opportunity to have scams, make money, putting medical workers at risk. At the time China was selling equipment at a third of the price, but it was not useable. The nurses spoke out in the news media saying that "the administration had made them disposable," that after seven months two thirds of the nurses still didn't have appropriate equipment.[1]

This was not only a criminal problem but also a business issue. There was a mask company, Prestige, that was located in Fort Worth, Texas, and whose CEO was Mr. Reese. He responded by hiring more employees and went from 60 to 260. But there was a problem during the Obama administration when the swine flu depleted the stockpile. Many of the N95 masks were expired, but Congress didn't provide them with the funds that were needed. Barack Obama spoke with the former president about the need for equipment with little success. And Mr. Reese told the administration that he could not live with a nine months contract and stay in business. What has emerged over the months was a battle between the administration's trade secretary plus a number of new providers that didn't deliver on time, and often doubled prices. The Defense Department was active in providing supplies, and Ford Motor began making ventilators. However, hospitals were desperately making calls for supplies.[2] Fortunately, now there are enough ventilators for the hospitals.

Meanwhile nurses like Brenda Halloum were caring for patients that were coming in at top speed with an unknown, and dangerous disease that she had never experienced before. She had worked with patients that have the Swine flu and Ebola, and so many different illnesses, but this one seemed like a baffling mystery. She found that they were all learning about Covid-19, continually as a new, inexplicable and very dangerous illness. It was like being in a new battle with the troops insufficiently prepared.

To begin with she was proning, turning the patient completely face down so that they could breathe, and then around, as well as bathing them because they were made unconscious given that the pain of ventilators was significant. They developed a technique on how to turn around 300 pound plus patients, and to keep them down while they were intubated, sterilized, and, medicated for 16 hours in a row. In addition, the nurses tried to maintain their oxygen level when the ventilators were not working as they should have.

In July they had many nurses that had worked with the coronavirus in New York, Tennessee, Florida, California, North Carolina, New Jersey, and Georgia. They were called crucials, also known as travel nurses, and were away from their families for six weeks with some of them staying from July until October. Some of the nurses were so grateful to have them on the staff. Brenda Halloum would take the time to feed them, and if one of them was leaving, she would give them a little gift to show her gratitude.

At the beginning of the surge, she would be in charge of just one ICU with twelve beds, but then she had to be covering all of their ICU Covid-19 patients, and was working with 24 beds because they had converted their day surgery into an ICU. They finally ended up with 50 beds. The unit she was in charge of was the 20-bed ICU, where she would see whether there were candidates that would be involved in proning.

Brenda had to schedule those, to see the kind of medications patients needed, whether they had received Remdesivir, a drug designed to fight other viruses, and what else could they do for them such as putting them on nitric oxide. Sometimes even after they were intubated, patients would not have enough oxygen, and needed supplemental medication. They were constantly deciding what they could do for their patients while they were facing so many other issues. This was before all the consequences of this illness were widely known. Faced with such enormous problems, the nurses were constantly asking themselves what else they could do for their patients.

Given the number of patients, the fact that initially they had no access to steroids and other medications now widely in use in her hospital, she was deeply upset for saving so few patients. Seeing so many patients die right in front of her is a burden she still holds since nurses spend so much time with their patients. Grief does not dissolve, but continues for a very long time, something people who have not lost loved ones may not understand. It needs to be shared and understood because feeling so alone with it is more than challenging. It was especially difficult because their patients were alone. All of the nurses were doing everything that they could possibly do yet were able to save very few people. They knew that they didn't have the resources they needed like the big hospitals, and that was also dismaying.

There was a time when they even had a doctor come down from California. He was taken aback and shocked by what he saw. By that time they were all doing rounds with the pharmacists, respiratory therapists, every medical person that would go to the unit. What the doctor saw was that hospitals and their addresses vary widely with some giving the best care available, and others struggling to meet their demands.

However, during the first weeks there were a lot of people that wouldn't go into the unit for a long time. Lobotomists weren't going there, the providers of ultrasound tanks, and people in radiology wouldn't go there. The nurses felt that they were doing everything at a time when they still needed masks and the proper equipment. The specialists would be there for a very limited time depending on how long they were exposed. It wasn't until the travel nurses, who were sent to help them by the defense department, that lobotomists, radiology technicians, and respiratory therapists entered the Covid-19 rooms. They then had the staff, and were able to do more proning than when they were alone. But for the nurses it wasn't enough, and they paid for it emotionally. The physicians who worked with them were also relentless while trying to understand this new and frightening disease.

Finally, they were getting the medications months later, but there were so many complications with this terrible illness such as blood clots. Some of their patients lungs were almost completely nonfunctional after months of being paralyzed and sedated, despite all the dialysis that they tried as well as the nitric- oxide, and chest tubes. It was very discouraging.

She still carries the weight of grief. When she came home after what she had seen in the ICU, she was very worried her children, wanting them to stay home after summer vacation rather then going to school. They watch the news on the television which she found discouraging. She is also concerned about her own children because one of them has mild heart problems so Brenda worries that if she has been exposed she is at high risk. Her daughter has a mild valve regurgitation which means that blood which usually circulates through valves in one direction, her daughter's goes in two. Since it is mild, her child's main symptoms are fatigue, but it makes her more anxious about her children's health. She is frightened and upset, and thus is now home schooling. She and her husband are trying to do whatever they can to protect them even though they wanted to send their children back to school. Many privileged people in our country are insulated, and are confident to make their choices in schools that are sanitized, and where students come in on different schedules in a hybrid fashion.

Differences With Her Community

When Brenda Halloum was shopping for groceries, she would meet people who went places, and would ask her why she and her family were the only ones that stayed home, not understanding the severity of the virus, and how it destroys people's lives. Her extended family had watched people on television going out, and they were annoyed that they couldn't travel. Moreover, they didn't realize why she came home so late, and had such long shifts in order for her to tell the patients' families that their loved one had died. It was very hard to explain this to the people she met, and to her extended family because they are not in health care, thinking that she was exaggerating. She found that it was very difficult to make people understand what she has been through without getting emotional about it. When she has the opportunity to explain her life in the ICU, she regards it as a way for people to understand what was happening in this difficult time because she has seen her co-workers tested positive who have lost their brother or mother only days after their test.

So far she has have been successful in not being infected. There were times after her shift when she would feel so exhausted that she thought that she was infected, and sometimes feels that it would happen regardless of her efforts. The nurses spend so much time in the hospital, busy with so many procedures such as intubating, and having so many patients on a bypass. She is at high risk of getting infected when a patient is on a bypass, and she is not wearing a shield. It took them a long time to figure that out and that is why so many staff members became infected. As a mother of five children and a wife, she is in a more than trying and dangerous job. When they would go into a room with a patient who is on a nitric mask with all the air escaping it puts them in danger.

On top of masks and eye protection, the nurses still had to get a total facial cover. The first time Brenda Halloum got tested was when she had an open heart patient. When she was prepared for a surgical procedure, the physicians discovered that the patient had tested positive. When she was proning a patient all of the air from the tube connected to the ventilator went to her face, because aerosols that carry Covid-19 are highly infectious. She had her mask, and her goggles, but didn't have the face shield that she needed to protect her. After that she wore her shield. She kept learning new things every day.

All three coronavirus units learned different things, and shared their experiences, learning from each other. These included how to make sure that patients get the ultrasound they need, that when a patient would complain about leg cramps, that meant that they had blood clots that would travel through their bodies. Brenda Halloum found so many things that could possibly go wrong, that happened with too many people. She saw people having their leg amputated or with filters because there were blood clots. It is such a complicated virus. She found that too many people think that the coronavirus is just like the flu. Many of her patients left the hospital without a limb, and most of them ended not coming out at all after so many months.

She became attached to her patients, and their family members she was in contact with. She was with them from the beginning. They may have started with a nasal cannula, the first type of oxygen they give when people are short of breath, and if that didn't work she would put on a mask, turn to a bypass, to putting a tube, and finally to the ventilator. Then when patients come out of it, she needed to inform them that they had so many family members that were affected, either close to them or scattered across the valley. They had lost so many members already because they have so many co-morbidities: high blood pressure, obesity, diabetes, and asthma. It wasn't until recently that the staff started giving them Remdesivir, and they were thinking that they should have a protocol for how to respond when they arrive, and do what is best for them faster. Remdesivir was approved by the FDA because it makes the recovery time five days shorter, 10 instead of 15, but it is not clear whether it prevents death.

Many patients came to the emergency room and tested positive, but they were not in respiratory distress, but overweight. Brenda Halloum thinks that before they are sent home, the staff should look at their history because she doesn't pass a week without having a patient like that, just 43 years old, but overweight. She found that if she didn't see them in the beginning, it was too late to help them. "A woman like that is not going to make it who is diabetic, hypertensive, obese and asthmatic.

When you look at her history, she should have received care immediately. It's so hard when it isn't considered on time." Ten days ago she would have gotten the Remdesivir, and convalescent plasma, which provide antibodies from people who have already recovered from the disease, instead of sending a person home. She believes that the staff should look at all of the risk factors.

She has a lot of responsibility, and cares deeply about every one of her patients. Her compassion has taken an emotional toll on someone like her who is working in what resembles a war zone. Brenda and the staff are trying to learn what they can from this illness and figure out what to do before it is too late. She wants new devices. They now have dialysis for the kidneys and there is something like dialysis for the lungs. She believes that we shouldn't have to go that far, but rather have had the appropriate treatment when it was sorely needed.

She thinks about our government that was so worried about the economy, and that if we had stayed in a lockdown, they could have avoided so much of this. Besides dealing with so many people dying, she feels that we need to move farther ahead with new treatments, and come up with new ways to confront this. She knows that for her hospital it's not going to happen very soon. In October 2020, they worked in a 20 bed ICU, but back in July there were almost 50 beds. So many of these people had such damaged lungs that they would have needed lung transplants, but fifty percent of them couldn't have them. So many hospitals in Texas are in the same situation.

Brenda Halloum is upset that we didn't have leadership in this country until a new president was elected in 2021. She tried to explain this to her children. She told them that this is a very bad example of leadership, that if we had a plan like we did for the Swine Flu or Malaria, we wouldn't be in this position. She finds it very sad that she has to tell her children, don't look at the president as an example, but as an example of what not to do. However, this is a learning experience for her children as well because they will grow up with more understanding. That kind of learning starts soon for young people whose parents work with coronavirus patients or who live in poverty, and it makes them stronger over time. Education happens in our daily lives not just in schools.

Good Days and Bad Days

When this country was experiencing a period of failed policies she was so courageous. She felt as if she were in a battlefield, and suffered terribly. Yet despite the grief for her dying patients, she educated herself about medications, and learned so much. Not many people understand that suffering is also a way of learning about life. For example, there is a new sense of gratitude when patients make even a slight progress, and gives one a perspective on what really matters in life, not just the small things. In fact Brenda Halloum not only experienced sorrow and dismay. She is grateful for everything she has learned during that difficult period when she cared for so many patients. Also, teachers have called her because they were so nervous about the coronavirus, and what it would do to their school. She replied that they were all in this together, that they would figure this out, that there will be some glitches, but it will work. The most important thing is to keep everyone safe. She remembers joking about it, how much of a nightmare it is, but telling people "we are willing to adapt with this whole situation."

Her children are learning along with her, and understand everything that she has to do. When Brenda Halloum comes back from work, sometimes they will meet her in the garage, and they'll see how tired she is and will ask her; *How bad was it, did you have a bad day, or how many people died today?* She is a wonderful mother.

People don't realize that she is facing a life or death situation. She is so fortunate to work with good people, and understands that there are good days and bad days. When she arrives, the first thing she does is to look at the board in order to see the people she will be working with. A nurse like Brenda Halloum needs to have a strong team to know what to do when things become difficult, and they have to move quickly. "To face a death together where there are not nice flowers, no gatherings for a funeral or mourning is deeply upsetting." For her there is nothing worse that seeing her beloved patients dying, withdrawing from her support, patients who want to be with their family members, but are alone, and just seeing them on FaceTime.

Unfortunately she has seen a lot of staff members who see their work as just a paycheck. Some of her co-workers saw a nurse who receives higher wages or has a higher ranking position and complained. During the most trying period some of them would refuse to go into the coronavirus unit. They would make up excuses such as the N95 didn't fit them or that they were concerned about their children. She found that they would treat the patients like pariahs. But she insisted that a nurse has to do a lot of critical thinking and to be constantly ready, telling them "it is not about you, but about your patients," that if they were having a panic attack they should still be with a patient whose life is at risk.

She would like them to get off Facebook, and Instagram. She doesn't have time for social media. Unfortunately she sees many of her co-workers who don't take their jobs seriously, and see the travel nurses making three of four times more than them with so much resentment and jealousy. She understands that the travel nurses are here as an extra set of hands that will help them to deal with all difficulties they are facing. She found that even when they are in the middle of a crisis, people can't stop thinking about money, but also think of what Brenda Halloum calls tiny things, and that she really had to snap them out of it. She told them to "forget about the paycheck, you need to get up, and get off your Facebook, and stop posting about your boss or whatever it is." She tells them to think about their patient that is in distress, that needs to go to radiology today, and that they need to be prepared for the worst.

Brenda Halloum needs to think about the back up for her back up. She is always trying to plan for certain things, trying to make it easier for the next time, to be prepared, whether it is having a test tube ready, or a central line for a chest set up. It will save her an extra ten minutes if she has to be gathering supplies, and she doesn't want to waste any time. While she knows that this was a learning experience, it was also deeply upsetting.

Then there is the issue of hiding one's pain. She has found that too many people want just good news, and not to be affected by what is happening around them. She can't talk to family or friends who don't want to know how she feels, and just how bad it is. They are more concerned with whether they can go out. Brenda Halloum can't tell them "ten people died yesterday, five aren't doing so well, and it looks like we are going to lose another ten today." She found that it doesn't matter to them, and that all they care about is whether they can't go out, travel, or go shopping. Their perspectives are in another dimension, and she finds it very hard to bear their conversations.

Her work is hidden and is important. People often ask her "How are you," which is only a greeting and not a real question. She answers, "I am," when people ask the usual question of "How are you?" whose meaning they do not understand. Her support is her husband and her children. She cries a lot, but the tears are way of lifting a burden. Having compassion can take a toll on nurses, on anyone who is caring for people who are going through difficult times. It not only happens in hospitals, but in so many working situations where people feel competitive, and instead of focusing on their work, they think about issues like power and money. Often we focus on success in a way that doesn't include accomplishments at work, or on the small things in our lives.

Nurse Brenda Halloum bicycles and runs a lot that helps her deal with pain. Running is a way of healing, and former veterans who have PTSD also run. She also does Yoga. She even grieves or feels stress on her days off, but her husband tells her to leave it behind her because she is no longer at work. However on her days off, case managers solicit her help even though she is not a manager. She receives texts with questions about what happened to a patient, and she responds by telling them what they could do. Her husband asks her why she is doing this on her days off, and she replies that it's important to share this whether she is working that day or not. She focuses on what matters, has a giving heart and a deep sense of commitment. She has found that helping in important ways gives her an uplift, and that feeling helpless exacerbates her stress. Not many people understand how giving of oneself is a source of deep satisfaction.

Brenda Halloum is working on the front line in the most trying place, with courage, compassion and, understanding. But she doesn't like the fact that people are posting themselves on social media as heroes, and believes that they don't need to be acknowledged or even to receive awards. When they left, some of the travel nurses gave her something to put over her badge that said Chaos Coordinator in the Covid-19 unit. But she has experienced joy and contentment with the work that she has accomplished for her patients, and is still dedicated to her job. She understands the oneness of our humanity. Not many people realize that suffering and joy are intertwined, and that her work is a profound learning experience.

PATRICIA RODRIGUEZ

In the Belly of the Beast

Patricia Rodriguez, who is a Charge Nurse of the Emergency Room at MacAllen Hospital, has found that it has been her most trying year in that position with so many people coming in with the coronavirus and dying. She is a very committed and sympathetic nurse who is used to saving people. When people came in who were so ill with the coronavirus she did all that she could for them with medications, and an oxygen mask. With so many of them desperate for air she found that it was like seeing a fish out of water. No matter what she did to stabilize these patients, they either died or went to the ICU to be intubated.

In one way she was fortunate, because unlike many nurses around the country who were either on strike or had quit their jobs for lack of PPEs and N95 face masks, she had a new N95 mask every day, enough PPEs, and she was tested. Although she had never tested positive, once she thought that she had covid-19 because she felt very tired, was short of breath and had a fever. She stayed in her room, her children were not allowed to come in, and her husband lived downstairs. She actually tested positive for typhus that comes from a tick bite, which can remain dormant in a person, but comes out when they are experiencing a high level of stress. It is hard not to think that one is infected when a person is working in the emergency room for so many hours.

Nurse Rodriguez found that everyone was susceptible regardless of their age. For example, some were athletes who were in very good shape. She read in the newspapers that people who are diabetic, have high cholesterol or heart problems were the most likely to catch this illness, but she saw that it also affected the young and the healthy. Months after her discovery, there was an article in the in the Journal of American Medical Association, December 2020, that had a section on the physicians' great concern for the rising number of young adults who are getting infected with the coronavirus.

She also found it so hard to see so much misinformation on social media that the coronavirus is a hoax, and that masks are not needed. She sees too many people who are so ill informed about the coronavirus whether because of ignorance or their political perspective. She wishes that they could see what is happening in the emergency room and the ICU.

Nurse Rodriguez remembers July as the most difficult time because that is when she treated many people with Covid-19 who were so ill that they were on the ventilator, and would be intubated. There were ninety patients with Covid-19 in the hospital in two days. All she heard was Code Blue every five minutes. She felt that it was like hearing gun shots. As a result, she still has nightmares about it, and her husband heard her cry in her sleep. She is overcome with grief and cries a lot. She didn't want her family or co-workers to know about that because in the emergency room she is seen as the brave one who can accomplish so much. She thinks that nurses are regarded as people who are tough, and that nothing bothers them, so she was afraid to show her emotions because people would think that she was weak.

Patricia Rodriguez and Dr. Vallejo became close, and shared their fear and concern when the cases were surging in July and in November. They were both afraid of how divided and uninformed a large part of our population is who don't wear masks, socially distance or even believe that the coronavirus is a threat. Despite the ignorance, and irresponsibility that pervade our country, she has dedicated her life to her patients. She is not only highly skilled, but treats her patients with kindness and a giving heart. How many people would continue a job that makes them cry so often or who would care for those in need. She is a different kind of heroine, not wanting to be one, only to help her patients, and give them her emotional support despite being frustrated by the wide spread lack of interest in the coronavirus or of people who are suffering from it.

On July 10th, Nurse Rodriguez was in charge of one of the biggest trauma rooms that the hospital tries to keep empty specifically for that or cardiac arrest. A sixteen-year old boy came in who was checked by his pediatrician the day before, and then sent home with a diagnosis of dehydration and vomiting. His father told her that he had been vomiting and having gastro intestinal problems for three days. She recognized these as symptoms of Covid-19 because young people have a lot of them that also includes nausea, as well as not tolerating food or liquids. She did CPR (chest compression) 40 minutes only to have him die; a beloved son, a football player, and high school student. She allowed the parents to stay there because they were so emotionally and physically drained. The mother who is deaf mute made the most devastating sounds. Patricia Rodriguez made the exception for their presence because they had been with him for those three days of his symptoms, and he was their only child. Her own son is 17 years old, and she kept thinking that it could have been him, a concern she lives with.

The following day she was with one of the emergency room doctors intubating a person, and there were a lot of people who were having difficulty breathing when she was called downstairs because they had two people with gun shot wounds coming in. They were both shot in the head by the same man who was beating up his own mother, events that occurred during lockdowns. Nurse Rodriguez is terribly upset by what this new disease is doing to people in a number of ways, seeing domestic abuse, the use of drugs, and the people who died from gunshots. In fact there has been a significant rise in the use of drugs since the beginning of the pandemic. It was a shock because she learned that people do these awful things when they are unable to leave, go places, and to socialize. She sees wounds in the emergency room that nobody sees; so many children who have been abused, including mothers and wives as well as people suffering, and dying from the coronavirus. After that she requested that her boss give her some time off because she was emotionally, physically, and mentally worn out. Nurse Rodriguez feels that she will always carry those two heart aching days throughout her life.

Throughout the pandemic she has been working days and nights although her hours are supposed to be from seven in the morning to seven in the evening. They were so short of staff as were hospitals throughout the country, but travel nurses came in help them. Yet, she would come home have dinner, take a nap, and go back to the hospital. She did that for quite a long time because she felt bad for the night nurses.

As a Charge Nurse she makes the decisions for the floor; receives the calls, responds to questions about what she wants them to do for particular cases in the emergency room. They also have to inform her when a patient arrives, and ask her where they should put that person. She also assists the doctors with some patients and then tries to get in touch with a patient's family members. She cares so much about her staff, that she supports them by working with them at night, often working 18 hours a day. She saw that everyone in her staff was exhausted, and didn't want them to have the same responsibilities as hers. Not only is she caring so much for her patients, but also about her co-workers.

Politicizing the Coronavirus Throughout the Country

Unfortunately like too many healthcare workers she is caring for people who are dying of the coronavirus yet who still don't believe it. Then there are the patients who are dying that caught the virus from a niece, nephew or grandchild who were at parties, and finds that is very difficult to deal with. Seeing the former president holding rallies without a mask with large crowds of people who were not wearing them, and cheering him upset her terribly, and also angered her. She wishes that he had acted like a leader, telling people to wear a mask, wash their hands, and stay at home if they are not essential workers.

Also she saw him as undermining our democracy and our values, thinking about the many thousands of lives that could have been saved. She worries about her own health. What gave her some relief was reading a story from Japan about how when broken objects are repaired with gold it gives the unique objects a history plus a chance towards beauty. That gave her another view of being heartbroken. She treats her patients like she would treat her family. One of her patients whom she cared for as if he were her son, told her that she had a heart of gold. What she didn't know was how from the beginning the Japanese government handled the virus with its own policies that had extraordinary success, and that the majority followed. It is the country of the G7 that had one in the fewest cases, and Germany also did very well with the coronavirus.

Not only is she angry at the former administration, but also with the governors of Texas and Florida. In the early stages of the pandemic governor Greg Abbott seemed more concerned about the economy, and not raising taxes. But when the vaccine for the virus arrived in December 2020, he was elated and finally spoke about the pandemic although it was a small number for the state's needs. What upsets her is that everything is open in Texas. There are so many people in stores, restaurants, and bars. She sees crowds everywhere as if we weren't living with an overwhelming problem in late November with more than 3,000 people dying everyday.

There are so many states that are against wearing masks such as Tennessee. In fact according to the New York Times writer, Nicholas Kristof, more Americans died from Covid-19 in nine months than in the combat of World War Two over four years, and sometimes losing more in a single day than perished in the Pearl Harbor and the attacks of 9/11.[1] She sees our country as lacking feelings of community and living with blatant selfishness.

Nurse Rodriguez is also upset about how Ron DeSantis, the governor of Florida, responded to the coronavirus. Many people including a man who sued the governor for his response to the spreading coronavirus, were furious about the 20,000 Floridians that died as a result. The governor's lawyers dismissed his case describing it as a form of empty political posturing that that requires political repercussions. Dozens of people told the Washington Post that the governor's decisions were more about politics, and lacked scientific evidence. DeSantis pledged not to institute a mask mandate or order lockdowns even as infections surged. In fact, he and his family were photographed without masks as part of a crowd at a high school football game.

On the following evening he held a large reception for state lawmakers at the governor's mansion despite warnings from federal health officials about large gatherings.[2] In addition, a Florida Scientist managing the state's coronavirus number was fired for insubordination by the Florida Department of Health when she refused to manipulate data to show that rural counties were ready to open. She also helped to build the statistics dashboard that revealed how quickly the virus was spreading in a state that did not mandate broad restrictions. On December 13, the Department of Law Enforcement arrived at her home with a search warrant, pointing their guns at her and her family.[3]

Despite her heavy schedule Nurse Rodriguez is aware of what is happening throughout the country. She wants people to open their minds, and realize that the world does not revolve around them, and that they need to think about the people who are suffering. She is so upset that they caused so much harm by not wearing masks or social distancing. She finds those behaviors as a lack of empathy, compassion or thoughtfulness. There is also a strong desire on the part of politicians to show that our economy is strong, that they are responsible for that growth, and will be reelected.

What upsets her is how many people come into her region to do their Christmas shopping, seeing a huge inflow of Mexican nationals who have visas. Many of them come to her town to spend their winter from a place that snows from October through March. When Texans go to Mexico to shop, and go to bars or restaurants, they come down with Covid-19. The CDC warned people not to travel to Mexico because of the high level of Covid-19 cases there. Yet the number of people from the U.S. visiting the state of Quintana Roo where Cancun and Tulum are located rose by 23 percent compared with 2019. One hundred flights were landing there every day in November. There was an art festival there with 1,200 people dancing, and eating in restaurants. The mayor of Austin sent a similar message, but it turned out that it not was recorded in Mexico. Days after the festival, there was a surge in testing requests from tourists, nearly all of which were testing positive.[4] However, Nurse Rodriguez decided not to visit her parents over Thanksgiving to ensure their safety even though it is only a two-and-a-half hour drive.

Nurse Rodriguez also worries that such a high percentage of people follows the former president, and keep calling our newspapers fake news. Those people get their information from YouTube videos, Facebook and Twitter. Recently the Federal Trade Commission sued Facebook, and there is an antitrust case against Facebook because it has more than monopolistic practices. It's also about the spread of fake news, conspiracy theories and its exploitation by authoritarian regimes.[5] Half of our country watches Fox News which doesn't provide real facts, but our President Trump turned away from its reporters because they disagreed with him, switching to a right wing news program Newsmax.

Nurses throughout the country are putting out videos to educate people, and some doctors and hospitals are putting articles in newspaper hoping to persuade people to wear masks, and social distance to protect everyone. Then there is Dr. Vallejo who educates people about the virus on TikTok despite his long hours of work. She finds that the emergency room is a war zone because, people are dying, and doctors are Coding so often.

Unfortunately she has seen that for a lot of people such as engineers, housekeeping employees, people who work in the cafeteria, and even some nurses are not upset. She finds it very sad that the patients who are dying are someone's parent, or child, husband or wife, and affects so many people. Even if it was a criminal in his last hours, nurse Rodriguez feels that they weren't born like that, and somebody loves them. Families matter in these terrible times, and some are showing so much initiative. For example in another state there was a wife who stayed outside of the window where her husband was ill with Covid-19, holding up a sign she wrote, "I love you." She thinks that to be a nurse you have to have a heart, and if someone who is dying doesn't make you sad, than a person like that doesn't belong there.

In addition to her concern for her patients Nurse Rodriquez feels anxiety, anger and fear. She is angry because so many people lack empathy, people that she thought were her friends stay out late at night drinking as if they forgot that if they are exposed to Covid-19 their families are too. She finds it very unfair because she is exposed, and is afraid to come home because she doesn't want her sons and her husband to become infected. She finds that people live only in the present moment as if there were no tomorrow, and that maybe there will be no tomorrow for them.

She sees people that are living in little bubbles. They tell her that staying home is a way of violating their rights, calling it freedom of choice, not realizing that when they infect people they really are violating rights. She takes on her co-workers when she sees that they are going places as if nothing was happening. Recently the Supreme Court made a decision that people have the right to attend religious services. There are many people who insist on doing so, putting other worshipers at risk. For example, there was a dispute between Orthodox Jews and the governor of New York, but the decision supported the Orthodox Jews. Some Christians travel to another state every Sunday so that they can attend a mass. In short, people don't want to change their lifestyle, and many are adamant about it.

She had discovered that it is the poor who have suffered the most from the coronavirus, and that a lot of them in the valley have used the emergency room as a clinic because they have no health insurance. She found it sad to see them with high blood pressure, diabetes, and Covid-19 at the same time. Many of them have left against medical advice, and she worries about them because she knows that they will die. However people who live in poverty need to pay their rent and feed their families. In contrast Europe where citizens pay high taxes, has universal health care as well as almost of year of unemployment benefits, which is social justice, not socialism as many people claim.

The Toll of Grief

Nurse Rodriguez remembers a nurse who dealt exclusively with patients who were raped. She could have retired because she was in her late sixties, but was devoted to her work. She was known for her work and was the first nurse to have that specialty in the Rio Grande Valley which inspired other nurses to follow in her footsteps. Unfortunately she arrived in the emergency room with the coronavirus, ended up in the ICU intubated, died a couple of times, was resuscitated with CPR, but finally died. There were so many other nurses that died in the hospitals in her area. "One is too many" she feels. They held a small memorial with her family at the hospital, and all of the nurses who worked with her. She found it a terrible burden, and worried that they will all end of with PTSD.

Also with new vaccines available too many people are against taking them, something that is not new. Previously some people thought that vaccines caused autism. The former president's supporters do not believe that it is safe or worth taking, a result of denigrating science and the facts about the pandemic. It is not an easy time to live in with the huge numbers of infected people rising. But nurses like Patricia Rodriquez never give up, and she has dedicated her life to healing, and caring for her patients, carrying a burden that too many people are not aware of. She lives with grief, and carries the images of the people she cared for and who died.

While we admit the reality of death and dying in our culture, we have yet to publicly to acknowledge the problems of our nurses who are dealing with so many deaths, and the importance of mourning. Nurses like Patricia Rodriguez spend so much time with pain and suffering. She feels the loneliness of her grief because in out contemporary society we consider mourning to be morbid, something to be avoided at all costs. However, it is the denial of mourning that is unnatural and unprecedented in history.

One nurse wrote a letter to her coworkers, including Patricia Rodriguez, about the depth of her sadness and emotional exhaustion.

"Walking down the ICU and every door has an isolation cart and a patient on a ventilator. To some people, it's just another hospital room. What I see is someone's wife, husband, their dad, their sister, or someone's child. Although we are all tired of isolation let me share my feelings that pour out when you watch: a wife pleading for her husband to stay alive, a daughter sobbing her eyes out on FaceTime, telling her mom as she is dying that she is carrying her first grandbaby knowing that she will never be able to hold that grandbaby, a son telling his dad how he made him into the amazing man he is as he takes his last breath, a mother watching through the window as her 38 year old once healthy child is Coded. These feeling weigh on you as you see that could be your loved one."

"I have held the hands of too many dying patients this year due to Covid-19. I have lost loved ones in my own family due to Covid-19. I have changed my life due to Covid-19. I worry every day about infecting my family and my babies, but my job is my passion and my other love. I was put on this earth to help people and I know that deep in my soul. For that I muster up the strength to push through with the weight of so many deaths on my shoulders. But I am TIRED. We are burned out in so many ways. My heart and soul hurts (who cares about feet). Death has become so UGLY. No one should die alone and we do everything we can as ICU providers to ensure that doesn't happen, but we are not their loved ones and that BREAKS me."

"I physically and emotionally could not do my job without the love and support of my colleagues and my support system. I love you all."

"Sincerely, A very tired healthcare worker."

The emotions associated with grief are very powerful and include anger, guilt, despair and sadness. Imagine how they are heightened when society denies their very existence. Not only do we experience intense emotions when we grieve, but in addition we are made to feel that somehow these emotions are inappropriate. Just when we are in need of social support we find ourselves isolated, without a common ritual or even a language with which we can communicate our feelings to others.

When asked to list the major emotions we experience in our daily lives, few people would include sadness or even consider it a powerful enduring emotion. On the contrary, sadness is often regarded as an unacceptable sign of fragility or vulnerability, but we are all vulnerable, not something that people like to admit. Nurses are living with death and dying, but often feel they should have been able to do more to help their patients. Yet it's the nurses that spend so much time with them, holding their hands, talking to them and seeing them end their lives.

The quest for meaning is also part of our journey through grief. As we struggle with our religious beliefs and our view of a just world, they may change radically like those of Nurse Rodriguez. Our belief in a benevolent Creator is often shaken when we ask ourselves why so many people are dying. We wonder why so many people are not spared this terrible illness, and ultimately death. We question the divine plan and think, unfair, unjust and more. Death causes us not only to examine our own lives, but also our place in the universe. Anger and grief are intertwined. These feelings are inexplicable and intense. Anger, guilt and sorrow are unpredictable, and do not necessarily occur in sequence.

Nurse Rodriguez has found that she experiences her emotions more deeply, and she cries more deeply. Every time someone is Coding for the coronavirus, she cries. She also feels joy more intensely, for they are also intertwined. People do not want to be vulnerable, but strong, but there are different kinds of strengths, like the sympathy and concern she feels for every single one of her patients. We have lost our social trust and ability to compromise that keeps our country united. Yet she is a very moral person who gives her life to her patients and her community. She lives with a lack of understanding of the coronavirus, and her non-stop stop efforts to heal her patients and their families. She feels that each patient is an important part of the world and should be treated as such.

HERRON ALVAREZ

Education and Advocacy

Herron Alvarez is a Charge Nurse in a Texas hospital near the Mexican border. His responsibilities include supervising a ward, delegating tasks among nurses, managing medical supplies and admitting and discharging patients. He began working with coronavirus patients since early May 2020. He was trained as an ICU nurse and was working in a step down unit that became another step down for the overflow of ICU patients. He was so terribly concerned about the spread of the virus that in addition to taking care of his patients, he began advocating for the nurses in his unit, and tried to educate them about Covid-19, which was such a new and unknown illness. He found it very hard to acquire his new skills, something he is proud of, but was also a source of concern because at the same time he was caring for Covid-19 patients who were critically ill, many of them dying.

In the early months, he didn't feel that he had sufficient expertise. He had only received two months of training while it usually takes about five months to train a nurse to work with coronavirus patients. Also he identified with his patients, and saw them in the context of their families; grandmothers, mothers, fathers, daughters, sons, sisters and brothers. The Rio Grande valley where he lives has a large Hispanic population, with multigenerational families living together, and thus in constant contact.

Nurses did not have access to the same equipment as physicians. They did have PPEs, but in the early months of the pandemic, they were told to reuse N95 masks several times in a row. At one point they tried to disinfect them with ultraviolet light before reusing them again. Unfortunately these masks are only useful for a single day, but despite this, they were told by the hospital administrators to keep using them for months. Naturally, they were concerned about their own safety, worrying about inhaling their patients' aerosols. Meanwhile he was carrying so many bodies out of the unit, and was concerned about the safety of his wife and children.

But there is one quality that nurse Alvarez brought with him to his new position—an independent mind. He keeps reading books about illnesses and newspapers to keep up with politics in the country. That led him to speak up to his supervisors when he thinks that preventive measures against the coronavirus are not being properly followed by the hospital. He also spoke up about the needs of his unit, the spread and the dangers of the coronavirus, and how he would like the hospital administration to respond. That is something is unusual for a nurse because some of them belong to unions or band together to discuss their problems, and share their concerns.

What upset nurse Alvarez the most were the poor relations existing between the nurses and the hospital administration. He was in touch with his immediate supervisors, but not with the executive officers, or the managers that worked just beneath them. Because of his concern with the coronavirus, he would talk to his supervisor and director about Covid-19, telling them that the virus was spreading, not only in the U.S. but also globally.

At that time, people who became infected on a cruise ship were quarantined off shore, and then brought to an army base for evaluation. One of them came to the hospital with a cough and shortness of breath and asked to be tested for the coronavirus. But at that time, the CDC guidance was that only people who had traveled abroad should be tested. Another patient who had attended a family reunion at an Air Force base in San Antonio along with people from the cruise ship checked in the hospital. She too had shortness of breath receiving the same reply with the CDC guidelines.

At that time, no one was wearing a mask and nurse Alvarez was very worried about that. He asked his supervisor if he could wear a surgical mask but he was told, "We don't want other people to be scared." During that time he was considered as an alarmist, but replied that it had nothing to do with fear, but rather with remaining safe, and being proactive rather than reactive like in so many other places. He added that to think that the virus was not going to spread, and that it was not in the U.S. or in Texas was being naive. With no response from his managers, he concluded that they probably had adopted the views promoted by Fox News.

Then, the hospital administrator summoned the nursing staff to a meeting, telling them that they shouldn't be scared. Nurse Alvarez was irritated because he felt that that administrator had no idea what it was like to work on the front lines. When he asked again if he could wear a mask, and had to insist before being finally granted permission to do so.

The U.S. Government left the decision about lockdowns up to the states, and Texas was late in imposing any in keeping with its well-known reputation as business friendly. It only took two weeks of protests outside Governor Gregg Abbot's mansion to convince him to rescind the order and announce his plan, "A Strike Force to Open Texas." That plan called for re-opening the economy in phases. The governor advisory board included restaurants associations and other business representatives as well as four medical experts who could have vetoed the decision. One physician worried that the state was not allowing enough time between phases of re-opening to measure the potential surge in infections. By Memorial Day, the state had re-opened stores, movie theaters, restaurants and more. As a result from May to late July, infections soared from about 1,000 to 10,000 cases a day. By late June, the governor shut down bars, and issued a mandatory mask-wearing order that saved lives in the following months. But, by November, he rolled back many of the lockdowns.[1] It was a precursor to his decision in February 2021 to end the statewide mask mandate and allow businesses to reopen fully despite federal advice against the states easing restrictions.

Also what was not disclosed until March 2021 was the case of a person who had flown from London to Dallas in December 2020 showing the symptoms of the B.1.1.7 variant, and who became the first documented case of that variant in the U.S.

In Laredo, Dr. Ricardo Cigarros challenged the governor on regional television. He made house calls to coronavirus patients, and was interviewed so often in an effort to inform the public about the dangers of the virus that the Texas Monthly called him the Dr. Fauci of Texas. He suggested that racism was involved in the way the crisis was being managed in Texas, and wondered why Republican state officials had allocated a higher level of vaccinations in counties whose population had a lesser proportion of Latinos.[2]

Meanwhile, as a Charge nurse, Herron Alvarez was working very hard to inspire his co-workers. He had two conflicting feelings, compassionate care, and working as a team, on the one hand. On the other he was upset to realize that the hospital executives were working in a safe location, unaware of what was happening in the wards and units. What he hoped for was some moral support for the difficult and dangerous work of the nursing staff. He was offended that it was the same people who told him not to worry about that dreadful illness and kept telling him that he was an alarmist for wanting to enlighten people about it. Before the coronavirus struck, he had created a Facebook channel to promote team spirit among the members of his unit, and provide them some medical information. He also invited doctors to participate in the project.

He even contacted a physician, and asked him to create a plan for educating people about the coronavirus because being uninformed made the nurses uneasy and fearful. Just a few minutes later, he received a phone call from an administrator asking him just what he was doing, and telling him that they shouldn't be disseminating that sort of information. He replied that he wasn't fear mongering, just trying to educate people so they wouldn't be afraid. And he added "if we learned more about Covid-19 and knew that we could wear surgical masks, it would decrease the amount of infections." He wanted his team to feel enlightened and empowered. He already had a list of questions on, topics the nurses wanted to learn about.

As the weeks passed and more and more cases broke out in the country, he bought himself a respirator mask. Unfortunately he was the only one wearing it at the time. He told his colleagues that they should wear masks because they were family members of the patients who came into the hospital, and few were covering themselves. Patients mingled with each other, and when they were coughing and sneezing, they were spreading the deadly virus. This was before family members were banned from coming into the hospital, and at a time when the danger of the coronavirus was barely understood.

At that time, people would ask nurse Alvarez why he was wearing a mask. He would explain the severity of the infections, but some argued that it was just fake news. Both his supervisors and his co-workers were questioning him. By the time they decided to wear respirator masks, the ones that used to be available at Home Depot for $30.00 were now selling for $200.00. He did some research and went through a Polish army supply company to get an army gas mask. His co-workers wanted masks that would be more durable than the N95 that needed to be changed every day.

There was also a lack of face shields, so he improvised one by placing a plastic covering over his head- band. Then he bought a pair of goggles, and even tried to use trash bags as PPE to limit his exposure.

When patient family members were again allowed into the hospital, although not in the Covid-19 unit, nurse Alvarez felt that this was a dangerous practice. Not only could they become infected with the coronavirus, but also they entered an area where the air was filled with infected aerosols. Nurse transport patients who cough or have shortness of breath must get Cat Scans so the virus can stay in the air for four hours because there is no air filtration there.

Nurse Alvarez also worried about asymptomatic visitors carrying the virus into the hospital. Even though their temperature was checked when they entered, and they had to wear surgical masks, many would remove them or let them slide down their face. He is so concerned that he thinks about what could happen, not just about what is taking place.

Members of the administration only responded to his concerns when they started running out of beds in the ICUs, and they had people waiting in the emergency room for at least one day before they could find a place for them.

As a Charge Nurse for his floor, nurse Alvarez is in constant contact with his patients' families. Since they are so close to the Mexican border, the community is mostly Hispanic and its older members are not bilingual. However none of the travel nurses could speak Spanish and so he is the only bilingual nurse there. At one point he had a nursing team with nearly 16 or 17 of them who needed orientation, to learn how to use their computers, how and where to get medications, and whom to talk to, Code Blue crises which happened so frequently. He also informed them about who was the most amenable physician, and who was the most difficult. Then he had to translate Spanish for every one of them. People don't realize that language and culture are so intertwined. For example in the Spanish culture, a person has to be more discreet, know how to say certain things, and even if the patient could speak English, he would want to talk to the Charge nurse to receive the information in a proper manner.

Sixty or seventy of the hospital core nurses resigned because of economic disparities. That can be upsetting. As a Charge nurse, Alvarez receives $30 an hour while a travel nurse gets $120, and with overtime, $180 an hour, making in a month what he does in half a year. These disparities are upsetting to him as he realizes that with a higher income he could pay for his mortgage and his children's college education.

Nurses around the country are quitting in droves because of lack of supplies, and the chaos in some hospitals. Even as late as December 2020, nurses around the country did not have adequate supplies and they had to buy their own masks and face shields. At that time, the surge of coronavirus cases was overwhelming the hospitals. Many them were lacking adequate resources and sufficient staff. Nurses were leaving their jobs because of their low morale, and because they were compelled to care for 15 patients instead of the previous number which placed an even heavier physical and emotional burden on them.

Few people around the country realize that nurses run the risk of getting infected by the virus, and some of them die. This is what caused some of them to move to less intense and dangerous work. Nurses and doctors are given priority to be vaccinated, and to some extent, this has improved the death rate. But still, in states around the country, nurses are going on strike because of insufficient safety protocols that cause patients with cancer or other illnesses to get infected with the coronavirus.

There was also the situation of the nurses lacking equipment in veterans' hospitals that prevented patients from receiving proper care. In one case, a BiPAP, oxygen mask, was missing, and the patient wasn't tethered to a monitor that could have alerted the nurses before he died. While every hospital in the country was facing a shortage of space and equipment for their patients, VA hospitals were did not have an effective system for tracking and delivering supplies. Also the VA was in the midst of a huge reorganization initiated by the previous administration that removed hundreds of jobs, and forced them rushing to hire contract personnel to help with the procurement of supplies. In so many cases, the vendors that were hired did not know what equipment was really needed, and were opportunists looking to make money while the nurses were told to keep using their N95 masks.[3] Then the nurses and physicians return from their demanding and compassionate work, seeing people in their communities going out in groups as if the coronavirus didn't exist and all was well.

The National Nurses United have been monitoring the nurses well being during the pandemic. They have documented the facts that hospital leaders undervalue the role of nurses working during the pandemic, and that they are getting unfair wages. That is a situation that upsets nurse Alvarez. Hospitals in the surrounding communities gave a $10 an hour raise to their nurses as a reward for their services during the pandemic, except for the one where he works despite the grave dangers to the nurses, and their family members involved in caring to coronavirus patients. Many nurses have been infected, and died from it as well as their family members.

Then there is the emotional and physical exhaustion, and the long-term psychological effects of nursing. Nurse Alvarez feels that doing so much every day for so many days in a row does change a person's attitude. This is because he cares so deeply about his patients, and because as a nurse, he spends long hours at his patients' bedsides while doctors and other personnel only visit them briefly. He has seen so many nurses suffering nervous breakdowns.

The National Nurses United has circulated the concept of the moral distress, and injury that they experience. They become real threats to their integrity when they know what the right thing to do for the patients, but the institutions where they work prevent them from delivering that treatment. That is something that nurse Alvarez experiences as he tries to give his patients the best care, but must work around the clock not only to have his managers listen to him, but to provide treatment from other departments. For many nurses, this affects their behavior and causes them to suffer PTSD, a condition that does not go away, and not only affects them but also their families. Sometimes nurses blame themselves for their patients' struggles to survive and for their deaths. Not only do they feel grief, but also shame and horror. Some of them feel numbed after so much exposure to suffering and death, just like military veterans.

Then there are also the long shifts without breaks, the lack of testing, the overwhelming workloads caused by inadequate staffing. Nurse Alvarez has seen all of that leading so many staff members to quit. Some hospitals are forcing nurses to keep on working after being exposed to the virus and testing positive because of a lack of PPEs, masks and face shields.

Anxiety and emotional exhaustion affect nurses who are forced to decide whom to give their attention to when they have too many patients. They do not have time to think about themselves as they go from one patient to another. Then they also worry about infecting their own families. Many nurses talk about having burnout, but the National Nurses United say that this does not represents the moral trauma, the low sense of accomplishment at work, describing it as an individual problem that can be solved with meditation, learning how to cope and self-improvement.[4] But there is a need for employers to provide social and financial support. Some hospitals do provide that support in states that are known for having the best hospitals and health care.

Taking Care of Patients

Caring for Covid-19 patients is an excruciating and a very disturbing experience as nurse Alvarez discovered. Unlike physicians, he found himself spending most of his 18-hour shifts with them and gets to know them intimately. When they stop speaking, he changes them when they have soiled themselves, something that he sees as breaking a boundary that they have maintained all their lives, in their intimate and personal space. He has a deep sense of compassion for them. And because he is so close to them, he knows when they realize that they are not going to survive. Some of them want to take off the BiPAP, and the masks that create a flow of oxygen into their lungs, the last step before intubating them. The BiPAP must remain for many weeks before it is possible to remove it which means that the patients are unable to eat. Instead they are injected with TPN, a liquid nutrition that bypasses the stomach and goes through their veins. It also means that they are deprived them of the satisfaction of eating something and of the presence of saliva which kills germs in the mouth and helps digestion.

Then there are the side effects on the patients of wearing masks for so many weeks, such as drying skin that peels off their faces with their noses and lids falling off. When air is pumped in for such a long time, the inner linings of their noses and mouths lose their moisture, their tongues become solid, and their throats are damaged. Nurse Alvarez saw patients chocking on their skin that had accumulated in the back of their throats because it is dried out. Some of his patients tried to take their masks off. Those who were successful died almost immediately because their oxygen level drops in just a few seconds. When this happened, the nurses restrained them and tied them down. Some patients became confused, took out their artery lines for their medications and die.

When a patient dies, the family members will question why the nurses didn't make sure that their loved one stayed alive. For nurse Alvarez, seeing his patients suffer so much is such a harrowing experience. He desperately wants them to heal, but being constantly at their bedside, he witnesses their suffering, and this is a traumatic experience. Living with so many deaths has taken a toll on him.

Nurse Alvarez has read a great deal about previous pandemics like the Spanish flu, the black plague, and the smallpox epidemic. Living through it is like being in another world, "It tears at your soul and pulls at your heart strings seeing people who are so sick, trying to help them, doing as much as you can." He thinks about how this is affecting their families, and how it changes the course of their own lives. He also worries about how this illness will affect his own family. It's such an overwhelming job to care for his patients that he doesn't have time to absorb what is happening at such a fast rate.

Another challenge for nurse Alvarez is getting the support from other departments in the hospital. He finds them very reluctant to assist his patients when they need their help. So another part of his job is getting the appropriate surgical care and intervention teams. It takes a lot of effort to persuade them because they are concerned about getting exposed to the virus. This may cause him to wait for days or even weeks before getting the proper support. He is also upset that while the U.S. is considered to be the world medical leader, it still lacks adequate health care resources for its people. Nurse Alvarez deals with so many patients who can die if they don't get the appropriate health care. Having the responsibility of somebody's life, he has to consider every factor. Yet he faces obstacles for unimportant reasons. Some doctors won't even see some of his patients because they are afraid of the virus. Being so dedicated to his patients, and caring so deeply about them, nurse Alvarez finds these issues very frustrating.

He has found that patient advocacy is extremely important because it is crucial to a patient's survival. If he did not speak for his patients, telling other departments what he is going to do and what he needs, so many of his patients would die. Once, he had an hour and a half meeting with a hospital administrator. In that meeting, he told him what he needed, and described how he often spent 72 hours a week with his patients. He also mentioned a number of things that were needed for his patients but were not being provided. All of this came as a surprise to the administrator because his office was on another floor, far from the coronavirus ward.

In January 2021, there was a Christmas surge of new patients, similar to what happened after Thanksgiving. They were not just elderly people, but also people in their forties and fifties who had to continue working. However, by then more patients were recovering so that they could be provided with oxygen upon their discharge rather than just dying. Unfortunately, they could not return to a normal life because they kept getting short of breath after walking just a few steps. They had to keep using oxygen from the machines in their home. Some patients returned to nursing homes or assisted living facilities. Others returned to multigenerational homes for cultural, and socio-economic reasons.

Some of the patients were so poor that they lived in sheds with their families, in just a single room with a bathroom in the corner. Nurse Alvarez worries about these people, and how to prevent the spread of the virus. He contacted social workers and case managers, but they were unable to help him. Some of the patients will be dealing with these problems throughout their lives, without knowing what is going to happen. He finds that prospect very frightening. He would like to see a more inclusive health care system, like the ones they have in Europe where everyone is covered, not just those who have private or employer provided insurance. Many poor people in the U.S. cannot afford good health because they can only eat cheap food that makes them gain weight, and predisposes them to become ill with diabetes.

Texas has the country's highest rate of uninsured adults and children, nearly 20% because it refused to extend Medicaid option under the Affordable Care Act.[5] Because coverage is tied to employment, the rate of uninsured had gone up during the pandemic as so many people became unemployed. This has exacerbated the large gap between rich and poor. Seeing this gap everyday along with the misery of those who become infected is heartbreaking for the nursing staff.

Nurse Alvarez is also dealing with new mutations of the virus that originated in the U.K, South Africa and Brazil, and that are even more contagious. In addition to caring for his patients, nurses like him are in a continual learning mode. Few scientists had expected the mutations to occur so soon. Early studies had shown that these viruses could have some resistance to the immunity people develop after recovering from the infection. In addition it is not certain that these are the only variants. So few countries, including the U.S., have invested in extensive genetic surveillance needed to detect emerging mutations. However by now, the Biden administration surveys 25,000 a week and MIT and Harvard are conducting sequence testing, along with the laboratories at Brigham & Women's Hospital. It is challenging to work in such a situation. Also, the virus knows no boundaries, so it will continue to affect us inevitably no matter where they appear. However, the new technology used to create the vaccines allowed them to reformulate vaccines faster than the more traditional methods.[6]

Vaccination rates need to be ramped up, and here again the protocols vary with each state. Nurse Alvarez was priority vaccinated, but he feels bad about the janitors who were told that they were not on the list of people who qualified. They are working in a war zone, with blood and urine everywhere, and although they now wear N95 masks, he would like to see them being vaccinated. He sees them as our silent heroes.

Given the surge of cases, nurse Alvarez doesn't know what is going to happen, and how long the pandemic will last. The many unknowns add to the nurses' anxiety when they realize that people in their communities have not changed their lifestyle. If they do think about the coronavirus, it's just when they learn of someone who has caught to the virus, and are concerned about their own vulnerability.

As the years pass, nurse Alvarez wants people to look back at the pandemic, and all the deaths that it caused. He also wants people to know that there is a meaning behind his team which he describes as so many events hiding behind the curtain, something that people who don't work in hospitals are not aware of. They may know the number of deaths, but they don't understand what is happening in hospital rooms with coronavirus patients, and how demanding it is to care for them. There is trauma and death everywhere. There are nurses like him who regard some of the treatments as a form of torture, with people being tied down, and masks on so tight, and the terrible side effects of intubations.

Nurse Alvarez has learned how to cope with grief since he experienced it in his early childhood. His mother died he was eight years old, leaving a four year old and a one year old sister. His father became very depressed and started drinking. It frightened him, but it made him stronger, and prepared to cope with this illness, and to understand our mortality. Then be became ill himself, and could no longer enjoy solid food, just drinking Ensure.

The way he deals with the burden of his life at the hospital is by taking a hot shower when he comes home, and thinking about all the things he is blessed with, his children, the woman he loves, the simple things of feeling that he is alive and can breathe. He has much in his life that he can cherish. He knows that he is working hard for his patients, giving them his 110 percent, and this makes him live in peace with himself.

Although nurse Alvarez is still young, suffering has been a learning experience for him. It has opened up his compassionate self so that he can share his patients' pain. Some people feel broken by it and some even commit suicide. But he calls suffering, "training of the soul, either you fail or you become stronger and it prepares you for life." He thinks that perhaps he would not have survived in this work had he not gone through such difficult times. Also he keeps taking time to read about what is happening politically, and feels that he has learned so much by expanding his horizons. He thinks about what happened on January sixth during the insurrection at the Capitol, that although Trump's presidential role is over, his ideas are not. He thinks about his legacy of the 560,000 deaths from the coronavirus, about the politicizing of mark wearing and the undermining of science. But he has found hope with the new administration, that there will be help with healthcare, preventive measures, getting the vaccine out, creating a competent scientific team that will help overcome these terrible times, and the domino effect of the coronavirus.

CATHERINE O'BRIEN

A Wider View of Nursing

Catherine O'Brien is a most unusual nurse. The time she spent caring for coronavirus patients moved her so much that she began to question how it not only impacted their health, but their daily lives and those of their families. She was concerned that patients in their early fifties who spent so much time in the hospital lost their jobs, their health insurance and important parts of their daily lives. She saw first hand the results of economic inequality, how we treat our immigrants, and ongoing racism. The issues she mulled over are ethical. She was also questioning the efficacy of our healthcare system. Even though she was only 28 at the time, she had an open mind that raised important questions as well as working with a caring heart.

She worked on a medical surgical floor of the hospital. When Covid-19 ramped up in New York City, Columbia decided to make the hospital a team to work with coronavirus patients because they are used to dealing with patients that have a number of co-morbidities. The Hospital could be first rate in managing those patients and the first ICU floor became solely for those patients.

However, in the last week of May the hospital was still lacking supplies for its health care workers. The nurses were encouraged to wear N95 masks as long as possible, to keep it in a brown paper bag, and put it in their lockers. In normal times they would take off PPEs before they left the room, and put it in the trash. If a nurse was in the green zone she could keep her PPE on and go from room to room. After a while donations of masks were coming in. The whole hospital became focused on Covid-19 from the end of March until July. The medical floor also worked with other illnesses, but not in the same room

Nurse Catherine O'Brien was working in same unit for two years. The nurses were working extra shifts, and a lot of overtime. Nurses spend 12 or 13 hours a day, so nurse O'Brien would feel guilty for leaving her nurses understaffed. She knew that her co-workers were exhausted, working more hours until they burned out, or became ill. Because it was so trying, some of them just quit their jobs. They had a group chat when there was a need for overtime, and those texts were coming through constantly. She knew that if she didn't take overtime, her co-workers would have more patients. Having patients to care for is a very trying workload, but the coronavirus brought them closer, although they were already in constant touch. They faced big challenges on her floor, because although she always had very ill patients, she hadn't experienced anything as demanding as the coronavirus.

What proved difficult was the number of times there was no place for the patients to go because the hospital was so full. The medical room is an acute unit, but step down is more acute, and then a patient goes to ICU. Nurse O'Brien worked with patients that needed step down care, but there was no room for them there. Thus the nurses remained with incredibly ill patients. That brought them even closer because they were in an unknown territory, and had to rely on each other just to get through the day.

The hospital wanted to minimize people going into Covid-19 positive rooms, a logic that brought the nurses to take on even more challenging work. They were bringing in the food trays so service employees didn't have to go in there, and asking their patients questions to avoid having social workers enter. As a result the workload on the nurses increased heavily which was one of the contributing factors for nurses feeling so burned out in the summer of 2021. Also the managers in the hospital were redeploying doctors, then putting extra work on nurses. There was some friction between doctors and nurses because the doctors were relying on updates from nurses, and they had to be everything for each patient.

Then as many nurses around the country, Nurse O'Brien found it difficult that the hospital was paying travel nurses twice as much as their own nurses' salaries for doing the same jobs. She had friends from nursing school who quit their jobs to become travel nurses because it's an opportunity to pay off their student loans. She is loyal to her unit and her co-workers, but annoyed at not being compensated as much for her work.

Despite being so busy, she noticed that the people throughout our country are not interested in the coronavirus. She found that upsetting because it could be one of them, and even if it wasn't she believed that they should care about the community, and not just about themselves. The hospital where she works is in Washington Heights whose community it serves includes a lot of immigrants, as well as diverse communities, which was another learning experience.

Becoming Ill With the Coronavirus

Unfortunately she became ill with the coronavirus. The hospital offered her paid time off for three weeks. When one of her co-workers had a Covid-19 patient whom they rushed into room, she may have forgotten her mask, and became ill five days or a week later. She feels that she was lucky because she is young and healthy. She also felt fortunate because she didn't have to use her vacation or paid leave time. She was given up to four weeks of time that was established for nurses who became infected with the coronavirus. Nurse O'Brien was very sick for two and a half weeks, and felt worse than she ever had before.

She lives in a small studio apartment in Brooklyn, and was so exhausted that it was a big effort to walk from her bed to the bathroom. It was hard to explain the aching and fatigue that she was experiencing. She was alone, but was worried about telling her parents because she didn't want to upset them. When she did give them the news, they were horrified. On the other hand, she felt lucky to work in New York City because while she was ill with the coronavirus she ordered groceries, and had them dropped at her door. But she found it frightening to be alone. However, she had worked with so many Covid-19 patients that she knew how to monitor her symptoms. She took her temperature every day, made sure to be hydrated, and did as little as possible. Also she checked in with her manager once a week to discuss her symptoms in order to decide whether or not she could return to work. And she thought "whatever will come, will come," and that she didn't have to worry about catching it anymore. She feels incredibly lucky that she didn't have any long-term side effects because she had worked with a young person in her early thirties who came in with blood clots.

When she returned, she had a patient who was close to her age, in her early thirties. Because she was sick she lost her job and her health insurance, an outcome so different from hers. They talked a lot about it. It broke her heart, and she was upset about seeing how people have no control of what affects their lives. Nurse O'Brien sees a willful ignorance with so many people, thinking that even if they get sick, it wouldn't be a big deal, but not thinking about what would happen to someone who had a different standard of living. For example, a man lost his job, but because he was undocumented, they couldn't put him in sub-acute rehab. His bill was astronomical, minus therapy, blood draws, and scans. She worried how he would survive. She thought, "We saved this man's life but to what end?" He has two small children, and sending him home altered the family's course. She felt that we have lost our sense of ethics. This is what keeps her up at night much too often. She works in a community with immigrants, and sees that they are the ones who work in low paying jobs that no one else wants. She sees that "We rely on them for all the services we love and take for granted," and finds it horrifying. That she cares is very touching because not many wealthy or comfortable people are concerned or want to know.

Patients Overwhelmed with Bills

Our hospitals are for profit in this country except for a very few that are dedicated to people who could not pay for their treatment such as the Boston Medical Center in Massachusetts. Too many people who had been treated for the coronavirus in hospitals live with the overwhelming problem of outstanding debts. Americans with serious illness usually face exorbitant and confusing bills, but many large health plans wrote special rules, waiving co-payments and deductibles for coronavirus hospitalizations. When doctors and hospitals accepted bailout funds, Congress prevented them from seeking additional payment beyond what the insurer has paid. Many patients found that these efforts did not work, and that bills can rise into tens of thousands of dollars, with too many of them winding up into debt. For ten months the New York Times tracked the high cost of treatment through a database that includes 800 medical bills submitted by readers. Those bills reveal that some hospitals are not complying with the ban on balance billing. Some are not applying the special coronavirus protections that insurances provided. Others are going after the debts of patients who died from the virus, pursing estates that would have gone to family members. Coronavirus patients are struggling with direct costs; money pulled out of savings and retirement accounts to pay for doctors and hospitals.[1]

Nurse O' Brian is also upset about racism. She thought of a young man who was morbidly obese, a big indicator for poor outcome of the coronavirus, and who lived in a poorer part of New York City that is a food dessert without grocery stores. She grew up in the suburbs where she could walk to three different grocery stores. He was only 39, but they knew he was in bad shape because his breathing was labored, and his heart rate was very bad. That was a sobering moment for people on the floor. They brought in an iPad so that he could say goodbye to his loved ones, and then he went to the ICU to get intubated. Nurse O'Brien thinks that it is wrong to regard people as responsible for the results of living in such difficult conditions. She sees that as a short sighted and self-righteous perspective. She thinks it is a prevalent line of thought in our country "Selfishness is when people say we want our freedom, meaning to go to a restaurant or a bar." She says, "there won't be a moral reckoning, if you can't find a small way to interact with one person that will help."

She has had a really rough year with her work because she has seen so much suffering that exacerbates the coronavirus; poverty, racism, and anti-immigrant feelings. She wanted to do one small thing for them, even if it was bringing them the kind of cereal they like. She found that it's the nurses who really care because they spend so much time with their patients that it wouldn't make sense if they weren't concerned about them, especially the ones that are in the hospital for a long time. Nurse O'Brien feels that if she could take something positive out of working with coronavirus patients it's the stories of people she helped in different ways; the younger man who lost his health insurance, the older man that they had to keep in the hospital. She views her job as an ethical and spiritual endeavor.

Too many people don't realize that illness is not just a physical problem but is also an emotional problem. People who are ill with the coronavirus face so many losses, not just in their finances, jobs, but in the daily toll of their physical abilities. A physician has written a newspaper article about the need to care for patients who may have recovered from the coronavirus, but suffer from PTSD, anxiety and depression. She added that mental health services were already insufficient before Covid-19, but rose with the number of patients who have recovered from the coronavirus with many lingering mental problems. This physician understands that patients feel they would rather not discuss issues of lingering pain so that their doctors and families believe that they are happy to be alive. While hospitals around the country are creating clinics for survivors of the coronavirus that are run by pulmonologists, they also include mental health resources for people suffering from anxiety, depression and PTSD.[2] As for the general public not many people understand that severe illness not only takes a physical toll on a person, but also a long lasting emotional and mental impact.

Moving On To A New Career

When she was in college, Nurse O'Brien studied Political Science, with Economics as a minor. She was interested in health care policy and then got a degree in nursing, which was also a learning experience about that policy. When she applied to nursing school she was so disillusioned with our health care system, and found that it's about money. As a result, she applied to a university in Britain, in order to get a different perspective because that country has universal healthcare. In the fall of 2021 she attended a graduate school in London for a Ph.D in global health policy.

In our difficult time of political polarization people are calling universal healthcare socialism and communism. Many of our contemporary republicans use the words "persistent socialism" for any policy that would help people who are less well off. Even out hospitals are acting like corporations. The biggest ones in Massachusetts have merged, and around the country big hospitals are buying smaller ones, so that competition has become an empty word.

What upsets her are the complaints about big government, and seeing universal healthcare as a form of socialism, not understanding that the countries in Europe that have this policy are democratic, and are financing that care with taxes. In addition, she sees too many people saying that they will be fine, but really don't care about what happens in another part of town, that the coronavirus has exacerbated the gap between rich and poor. Also she regards many people as self-righteous, believing that the previous administration did everything right. "There were too many people having to pretend that it wasn't happening, and then finding ways to justify over half a million deaths."

The healthcare system had problems for decades, lacking federal standards and federal funding for a number of issues including genomic sequencing that was initiated, although at a low rate, by President Joe Biden. There is also a need for incident reporting and establishing federal standards. The problem of cyber attacks that became public when the Colonial Pipeline became widely known also created major health problems for hospitals after attacks on their systems. For example California's Scripps Health was just starting to serve patients after going dark for most of the month. In 2020, 2021, cyber criminals shifted their focus to bigger health care targets that have failed to implement basic security practices. Recovering from these attacks is much more difficult than paying a ransom, decrypting data and resuming business. Attacks have left hospitals struggling for weeks and even months. The cyber security firm Emisoft found that 21 attacks took place on U.S. health care providers, affecting about 50 facilities. The previous year 80 attacks took place around 560 facilities that included 400 locations and that were part of the attack on Universal Health Care Services in the Fall of 2020.[3] This is a difficult time to acquire federal funding, and it puts healthcare workers and their patients in a terrible position.

Also, not many people are aware of the connection between climate change and medical care. Climate change affects people's lungs and makes them more vulnerable to the coronavirus, but hospitals are also dealing with climate change such as wildfires or flooding that is putting them in peril across the country. Changes to create resilience include moving technical equipment from basements where floodwater could damage it, organizing patient transfers in advance of catastrophes, improving energy efficiency and air filters. For example, The Boston Medical Center has lowered its energy use by 40 percent, and reduced its greenhouse gas emissions by 90 percent while caring for more patients. It also created a rooftop garden that grows about 6,000 pounds of food a year for its food pantry inpatient meals, a hospital based farmers' market and a bio-digester that converts food waste into water.[4] During heat waves and fire seasons power can go out or electric utilities may shut off power to avoid fires or creating wide blackouts which means hospitals have to rely on generators.

In New York City, New York University's Langone Health built a cogeneration plant for electricity and heat plus steam turbine power for air conditioning. The cogeneration plant was in place before Hurricane Sandy. During the storm, floodwater reached the lower floors of the hospital, leaving millions of gallons of contaminated water. More than 300 patients had to be evacuated. The hospital was closed for two months after the storm. There are now flood barriers around the campus in order to protect it against a storm surge seven feet above the level caused by Hurricane Sandy.[5] Not many people think about the connection between climate change, hospital operations, and medical care.

As of June 2021, Nurse O'Brien had only had a few coronavirus patients on her floor, but there were incredibly short-staffed. Yet many nurses left the profession to take time off because they were tired of the pressures, wanting to spend time with their families or go to a different kind of job because of their exhaustion and the tension of working such long hours with so many patients to care for. New York State Union of nurses had been trying to make a difference. Unfortunately there were hiring freezes on her floor because they had less money. As a result the hospital was hiring graduates, but they required training. Then they also were hiring travel nurses to fill the gap that irritated her because of the decline in funds. She felt bad about leaving, and that even though she was going to graduate school to study health policy, they were short of another nurse.

When she has received her degree, she would like to be professor. She sees so many problems in our healthcare systems that she want to learn ways to make the changes we so need that are "transformative instead of putting on band aids," hoping that they will survive.

Nurse O'Brien is very concerned about the current situation in our country that has evolved during the Trump presidency. She found that it has emboldened people to subvert peoples rights such as the new voting laws that have been passed in a number of states like Texas and Utah, limiting the hours when people can vote and affecting our black, Hispanic and impoverished populations. Republicans talk about any help for the poor and needy as socialism or communism. She found that it is not possible to talk people about political issues.

She wants to teach health policy because she is concerned about health care inequities. She has seen too many people who don't have access to health care. She has also witnessed that parts of the staff are saying that it's the patients fault for being sick, overlooking the fact that they live in poverty. One of her goals is to increase access to healthcare in the U.S. A person can walk into an ED and be seen, which doesn't make it accessible health care. She believes that we should be providing preventable health care so that people can walk into in a doctor's office. Growing up in a middle class family, she had preventative healthcare such as yearly check ups covered by her insurance, and had hearing and vision screening every year. Access to healthy fruit and vegetables, and extracurricular activities is an important source of health.

But in U.S. health care is so expensive and so difficult to access. Finding providers in a network can be an absolute nightmare. People aren't going to see doctors regularly that would prevent them from getting sick. Instead they are going to emergency rooms because they have no other option. When she checked patients' finger tips for oxygen, or the AIC, an indication of diabetes, the level of a person's blood sugar, these are people who are obese, and often can't afford good nutrition. She thinks that we need to be concerned about that and to keep an eye on these patients. Because we haven't provided that from the beginning, they are coming in when they are seriously ill. For example too many people come into emergency rooms because that is the only recourse they have to get help for health problems. Then they are put on a very expensive medication that many of them are unable to afford. She has found that staff members feel that they should know that their insulin is important. Patients certainly know that, but are unable to afford it. They have to make a decision between feeding their families and buying the much-needed medication.

That is proven by a five-year study by the Boston Foundation that revealed that housing instability affects the health of low-income Boston area residents. It's Health Starts at Home initiative provided funding for four local organizations that work on housing and health care. They hired housing counselors to connect struggling families with resources that were available in the community and helped isolated families to learn about support options. The project has been in place for five years, and in a number of cases provided financial support for housing. Seventy eight percent of the families were Hispanic or Black. The studies showed that the percentage of families worried about eviction or foreclosure dropped significantly, and that children's emergency room visits were nearly cut in half.[6] Not many people realize how daily stress causes illness as well as feeling isolated without any personal support. The necessity of preventive care has been one of nurse O'Brien's biggest concerns.

What bothers her about healthcare in general, is the response of physicians who say "We told you what to do," to patients. The system doesn't take into account how broken it is. She has seen that in general, patients are pushed out because they have more patients that need to come in. She is upset that we don't have enough doctors, and found that "we are burning the candle at both ends, and that we don't see that the way we are operating is going to lead to a mass exodus for people from the health care system. We are tired of trying so hard swimming upstream." Eventually you reach a point where you feel that you can't do this anymore. She has seen it with the nurses and PA's who are exhausted. People in the community don't realize what is happening in hospitals, but are only concerned about being able to go to a restaurant.

Nurse O'Brien worries about our political and social system. She found that people now seek out reinforcement as opposed to facts. If a person already has some thoughts about what is happening, they will seek out information that reinforces and validates it as opposed to being critical. She is also concerned about the far left that wants immediate solutions, and the far right's scare tactics.

She has worked as nurse in homeless shelters. When an uncle told her "I don't know how you work with these junkies," she responded, "If you read these people's stories you have no right to judge anyone of them. The fact that they are alive and doing what they need to do and based on the history they had it's a miracle." She thinks that it's wrong to think that a person's wealth is more important than the right to survive, and cares so much about human rights. She has brought a wide and inspired vision to her time in nursing that will bring her to another way of making a difference.

HEALING

Reading the news about the number of people
infected with covid-19, the rising curve
of deaths among the people who
were the most vulnerable; minorities

who did the *essential work*, and their zip codes,
immigrants living in apartments so crowded
they rented their beds while they worked
their night shifts. And in this country

which is already so divided, some of us
have put our hearts and minds on hold
because they have higher needs; businesses
shut down, restaurants, stores, and bars

needing to open, some marching for *freedom*
with their rifles. But then there are the nurses
and physicians, working around the clock,
holding their patients' hands, putting

their own lives at risk, joining our
grieving, reminding us that we need to reach
out to one another, that caring for
each other is a higher form of healing.

—Marguerite Guzmán Bouvard

NOTES

Introduction

[1] Angus Chen, "Genetic 'Fingerprints' Suggest Superspreader Biogin Conference Seeded 40% of Boston Coronavirus Cases," WBUR, August 25, 2020.

[2] National Nurses United. 2021. (https://www.nationalnursesunited.org).

[3] Kent Bab, "As Thousands of Athletes Get Coronavirus Tests, Nurses Wonder: What About Us?" *The Washington Post*, November 27, 2020.

[4] Yann Kebbi, "Nobody Accurately Tracks Health Care Workers Lost to COVID-19," Special to *ProPublica*, August 22, 2020.

[5] Peter Goodman, "Covid Overload Pushes Hospitals Across the Nation Closer to Breaking Point," *The New York Times*, November 28, 2020.

[6] "In Harm's Way: Fighting the Summer Surge," *The New York Times*, August 1, 2020.

[7] Vanessa Romo, "NYC Emergency Room Physician Who Treated Coronavirus Patients Dies by Suicide," WBUR, April 28, 2020.

[8] Adam Stariano, "Doctors Do Battle with False Information," *The New York Times*, August 17, 2020.

[9] William Wan, "Burned Out by the Pandemic: 3 in 10 Health-Care Workers Consider Leaving the Profession," *The Washington Post*, April 22, 2021.

[10] Chavi Eve Karkowsky, "Women in Health Care Without Schools Will Quit," *The Washington Post*, July 26, 2021.

[11] Colin Binkley, "School Survey Shows 'Critical Gaps' for In-Person Learning," *The Washington Post*, March 24, 2021.

[12] Dina Temple Raston and Tim Mak, "HHS Renews $10.2 Million Contract for Controversial Covid-19 Data-Tracking Company," WBUR October 2, 2020.

[13] Sheryl Gay Stolberg, "Health Experts Raise Alarm Over Federal Rules on Hospital Data," *The New York Times*, August 12, 2020.

[14] William Wan, "Burned Out by the Pandemic: 3 in 10 Health-Care Workers Consider Leaving the Profession," *The Washington Post,* April 22, 2021.

[15] Ibid.

[16] Ibid.

[17] Apoorva Mandaville, "Journals Understate Systemic Racism," *The New York Times*, Science Times, June 8, 2021.

[18] Jane Greenhalgh and Patti Nighmong, "The Majority of Children Who Die of Covid-19 are Children of Color," WBUR, September 16, 2020.

[19] This article is by Eddie Burkhalter, Izzy Colón, Brendon Derr, Lazaro Gamio, Rebecca Griesbach, Ann Hinga Klein, Danya Issawi, K.B. Mensah, Derek M. Norman, Savannah Redl, Chloe Reynolds, Emily Schwing, Libby Seline, Rachel Sherman, Maura Turcotte and Timothy Williams, "Incarcerated and Infected: How the Virus Tore Through The US. Prison System," *The New York Times,* April 10, 2021.

[20] Miriam Jordan, "U.S. Must Release Children From Family Detention Centers, Judge Rules," *The New York Times*, June 26, 2020.

[21] Lylla Younes, "New Studies Show Disproportionate Rate of Coronavirus in Polluted Areas," *ProPublica*, September 11, 2020.

[22] "3C Epiphany," *The Economist*, December 12, 2020.

[23] Li Yuan, "The New World." *The New York Times*, Business, January 5, 2021.

[24] PBS Frontline, February 2, 2021.

[25] "Lab leaks of Virus," *Politico Nightly*, May 19, 2021.

[26] Dhruv Khuuar, India's Crises Marks a New Phase in the Pandemic, *The New Yorker*, May 15, 2021.

[27] "The Geometry of the Pandemic," *The Economist*, July 25, 2020.

[28] Rebecca Hersher, Nathan Rott, and Lauren Sommer, "Everything is Unprecedented. Welcome to Your Hotter Earth," WBUR, August 26, 2020.

[29] Henry Fountain, "Lower Humidity Presents Fire Risk for Drier Southwest," *The New York Times*, June 23, 2021.

[30] John Schwartz, "Wilting Heat, Intensified by Climate Change," *The New York Times*, July 16, 2020.

[31] Laurel Wamsley, "Haze Spreads Across the US As Wildfires Continue to Burn," WBUR, September 16, 2020.

[32] Cleve R. Wootson and Karin Brulliard, "Coronavirus spikes in Oregon as residents evacuate wildfires,"*The Washington Post*, September 19, 2020.

[33] Lisa Song & Lylla Younes, "The EPA Refuses to Reduce Pollutants Linked to Coronavirus Deaths," *ProPublica*, October 20, 2020.

[34] John Dillo, "Shelter from the Climate Storm? Experts Say Vermont Needs to Prepare for Climate Migration." Vermont Public Radio, April 21, 2021.

[35] James Barron, "Coronavirus Update," *The New York Times,* February 16, 2021.

[36] Abraham Lustgarten, "Climate Change Will Force a New American Migration," *ProPublica*, September 15, 2020.

[37] David Quammen, *Spillover*, New York: W.W. Norton & Company, 2012.

[38] Ferres Jabr, "How Humanity Unleashed A Flood of New Diseases," *The New York Times*, June 25, 2020.

[39] Tara Parker Pope, "Stories Behind the Guises of Covid-19," *The New York Times*, August 1, 2020.

[40] William Stone. "Clots, Strokes and Rashes. Is Covid-19 A Disease of The Blood Vessels?" WBUR, November 5, 2020, in partnership with Kaiser Health News.

[41] Dr. Robert Klizman, "Our Next Crisis Will Be Caring for Survivors of Covid-19." *The Washington Post*, June 4, 2020.

[42] Lenny Bernstein,"'Nobody Has Any Clear Answers for Them'; Doctors Search for Treatments for Covid-19 Long-haulers," *The Washington Post*, October 16, 2020.

[43] Pam Belluck, "First a Mild Case, Then a Deluge of Misery," *The New York Times*, March 24, 2021.

[44] "And Now for the Aftershock," *The Economist*, May 1, 2021.

[45] Chico Harlan and Stefano Pitrelli, "Italy's Bergamo is calling back coronavirus survivors," *The Washington Post,* September 8, 2020.

[46] Emma Goldberg, "The Mental Toll of an Illness That Won't Go Away," *The New York Times*, September 8, 2020.

[47] Brady Dennis, Chris Mooney, Sarah Kaplan, and Harry Stevens, "Scientists Have a Powerful New Tool for Controlling the Virus: Its Own Genetic Code." *The Washington Post*, October 13, 2020.

[48] Mike Baker, "Throwing Up Their Hands and Taking off Their Masks," *The New York Times,* November 2, 2020.

[49] Sheryl Gay Stolberg and Carl Zimmer, "Highly Contagious Variant Is Dominant in New Cases, CDC Director Says," *The New York Times*, April 8, 2021.

[50] Jennifer B. Nuzzo and Emily N. Pond, "Covid Vaccines Aren't Enough. We Need More Tests," *The New York Times*, March 13, 2021.

[51] Noah Weiland, "Emails Describe Effort to Muzzle Directors at CDC," *The New York Times*, September 19, 2020.

[52] Editorial, *The Washington Post*, August 7, 2020.

[53] "Widely Available Steroids Reduce Mortality in Severely Ill Covid-19 Patients, Research Found," *The Guardian*, September 2, 2020.

[54] Bianca Motley Broom, "To Save Lives, My City Ordered Locals to Wear Masks. The Government Blocked Us," *The Washington Post*, July 24, 2020.

[55] Lisa Creamer, "Starting Aug. 1, Many Travelers To Mass. Must Quarantine For 14 Days, Or Test Negative," WBUR, July 24, 2020.

[56] Annie Karni, "U.S. Opens Ad Campaign to Combat Hesitancy," *The New York Times*, April 2, 2021.

[57] Apoorva Mandavilli, "'Herd Immunity' Dims As Vaccinations' Pace Begins to Slow Down," *The New York Times*, May 3, 2021.

[58] Jonathan Wolfe, "Coronavirus Briefing: What Happens Today," *The New York Times*, April 8, 2021.

[59] Fenit Mirappil and Ashley Cusik, "When delta strikes: Latest coronavirus surges grow faster, hits record heights in Louisiana, Florida," *The Washington Post*, August 3, 2021.

[60] Rick Rojas, "Demand for Shots Quadrupled," *The New York Times*, August 5, 2021.

[61] Roni Caryn Rabin, "'Younger, Sicker, Quicker': Doctors See Change in Covid Patients," *The New York Times*, August 4, 2021.

[62] Maggie Astor, "Covid Survivors Emerge as Political Activists," *The New York Times*, March 18, 2021.

[63] Stephen Engelberg, "Why We Are Publishing the Tax Secrets of the .001%," *ProPublica,* April 2, 2021.

[61] Carl Zimmer, "Researchers Are Hatching a Promising Low-Cost Coronavirus Vaccine," *The New York Times,* April 6, 2021.

[65] Carl Zimmer, "German Company's Vaccine Could Offer Hope to Hard-Hit Countries," *The New York Times*, May 6, 2021.

[66] "The Insufficient Miracle," *The Economist*, May 15, 2021.

Dr. Jorge Mercado

[1] Marisa Taylor, "Exclusive: U.S. axed CDC expert job in China months before virus outbreak," Reuters. 3/22/2020.

[2] Frontline, June 16, 2020.

[3] Josh Rogin, *Chaos Under Heaven: Trump, XI, and the Battle for the 21st Century.* (Boston: Houghton Mifflin Harcourt, 2021), 255-269.

[4] Ibid.

[5] Cory Deburghgraeve as told to Eli Saslow, "Voices from the Pandemic," *The Washington Post*, April 5, 2020.

Dr. Martin Schwarcz

[1] Marguerite Guzmán Bouvard, *Social Justice and the Power of Compassion*, (New York: Rowman & Littlefield, 2016), 109.

[2] Anabel Munoz, "Medical Expert Peter Hotez Describes 'Historic Decimation' of Latinos by Covid-19," ABC, October 1, 2020.

[3] Dara Lind, "Hospitals Are Suddenly Short of Young Doctors — Because of Trump's Visa Ban", ProPublica, July 17, 2020.

Dr. Eduardo Mireless

[1] James Hamblin, "A Covid-Vaccinated Summer Could Be Wonderful," *The Atlantic*, February 19, 2021.

[2] Caroline Chen, "Fauci: Vaccines for Kids as Young as First Graders Could Be Authorized by September, " *ProPublica*, February 11, 2021.

[3] "Briefing: Making Vaccination Work," *The Economist*, February 13, 2021.

[4] Mike DeWine, "A Vaccine Lottery Can Work," *The New York Times*, May 27, 2021.

[5] Cleve R. Wootson, Jr. and Frances Stead Sellers, "Biden's Vaccine Push Runs into Distrust in the Black Community," *The Washington Post*, February 13, 2021.

[6] Lyn Chutel and Marc Santora. "Posing Global Threat, Variants Spread Where Vaccines Have Not," *The New York Times*, February 1, 2021.

[7] *Politico Nightly*, March 12, 2021.

[8] Ishaan Hardoor, "The Pandemic Leads to New Forms of Inequality," *The Washington Post*, February 19, 2021.

[9] Miriam Berger, "Global vaccine inequality runs deep. Some countries say that intellectual property rights are part of the problem," *The Washington Post*, February 20, 2021.

[10] Sheryl Gay Stolberg and Michael Crowley, "U.S. Takes Steps to Use Vaccine for Diplomacy," *The New York Times,* March 13, 2021.

[11] Patrick Kingsley, "Israeli Vaccines go to Far-Off Allies Before Palestine," *The New York Times*, February 24, 2021.

[12] Lazaro Gameo and Alexandrea Symondo. "Global Virus Cases Reach New Peak, Driven by India and South America," *The New York Times*, May 1, 2021.

[13] Claire Parker, Paul Scherm, and Sean Sullivan. "India Sets Another Daily Coronavirus Record; U.S. Pledges Help," *The Washington Post*, April 26, 2021.

Dr. Federico Vallejo

[1] Reed Abelson, "Doctors Are Calling It Quits," *The New York Times*, November 16, 2020.

[2] Jeneen Interlandi, "Now the President and the Frontline Workers Have Something in Common," *The New York Times*, October 3, 2020.

[3] Mike Hixenbaugh, NBC News, and Perla Trevizo, *The Texas Tribune* and *ProPublica*, "Texans Recovering from COVID-19 Relied on Machines to Help Them Breathe. Then the Power Went Off," March 9, 2021.

[4] Erin Cunningham, "Texas Gov. Greg Abbott Issues Order Banning 'Vaccine Passports' in the State," *The Washington Post*, April 6, 2021.

[5] Alan Feuer, "Capitol Rioter Traveled from Towns Where Fear of Racial Change Prevails," *The New York Times*, April 7, 2021.

[6] Robert Barnes, "Supreme Court Vacates Ruling Barring Trump from Blocking Twitter Critics, Saying Case is Moot," *The Washington Post,* April 5, 2021.

[7] Ann Goldstein, *"*Should Health-Care Workers Be Required to Get Coronavirus Shots? Companies Grapple with Mandates," *The Washington Post*, April 5, 2021.

Dr. Susan Ly

[1] Carl Zimmer, "Variant First Seen in U.K. is spreading Rapidly in US., Study Finds," *The New York Times*, February 8, 2021.

[2] Joel Achenbach and William Booth, "Worrisome Coronavirus Mutation Seen in U.K. Variant and in Some U.S. Samples," *The Washington Post*, February 2, 2021.

[3] Isaac Stanley-Becker, "Anti-vaccine Protest at Dodger Stadium was Organized on Facebook, Including Promotion of Banned 'Pandemic' Video," *The Washington Post*, February 1, 2021.

[4] Nurith Carlson and Ruth Talbot, "Actual Number of Active Cases Infected Likely 10 Times Worse Than You Thin," WBUR, January 6, 2021.

[5] Andrew Jacobs, "One Year In, Pandemic Pushes Health Care Workers to the Brink," *The New York Times*, February 5, 2021.

[6] Margaret Sullivan, "These Local Newspapers say Facebook and Google are Killing Them. Now They're Fighting Back," *The Washington Post*, February 4, 2021.

[7] Lynn Jolicoeur, "Mass. Physicians Call on State To Address ER 'Boarding Of Patients' Awaiting Admission," WBUR, February 2, 2021.

[8] Lisa Mullins, Lynn Jolicoeur, "Mass. Psychiatrists Concerned About Increase in Suicidal Thoughts," WBUR, March 25, 2021.

[9] Andrew Jacobs, "One Year In, Pandemic Pushes Health Care Workers to the Brink," *The New York Times*, February 5, 2021.

[10] Gaynell Paul Matherne and Emily Jane Orr, "Translating Personal Tragedy into Action; Starting the Lorna Breen Heroes Foundation", (*Charlottesville, VA: Darden Business Publishing*, October 30, 2020).

[11] Abby Ellen, "Faced with Burnout Doctors Recommend Caring for Themselves," *The New York Times*, February 2, 2021.

[12] Alec Macgillis, "The Lost Year: What the Pandemic Cost Teenagers." *ProPublica*, March 8, 2021.

[13] Apoorva Mandavelli, Kate Taylor ,and Dana Goldstein, "CDC Offers Paths to Reopening Schools," *The New York Times*, February 13, 2021.

[14] Emma Goldberg, "Doctors in a Bind," *The New York Times*, February 23, 2021.

Dr. Edy Kim

[1] Michaeleen Doucleff, "Why Scientists Are Very Worried About the Variant from Brazil," NPR, January 27, 2021.

[2] "Variants on a Theme of Disaster," *The Economist*, March 24, 2021.

[3] Brady Dennis, Chris Mooney, Sarah Kaplan, and Harry Stevens, "Scientists Have a Powerful New Tool for Controlling the Coronavirus: Its Own Genetic Code," *The Washington Post*, October 12, 2020.

[4] Apoove Mandaville and Benjamin Mueller, "Virus Variants Threaten to Draw Out the Pandemic Scientists Say." *ProPublica*, April 4, 2021.

[5] Genomic Surveillance Dashboard, March 14, 2021 (https://stacks.cdc.gov/view/cdc/104210).

Sarah Ghozayel

[1] Latishia Beacham, "Florida Sets Another High and Other States See Infections Rise," *The Washington Post*, July 2, 2020.

[2] Moriah Balingat, "Florida Orders Schools to Reopen Even as Virus Cases Soar," *The Washington Post*, July 6, 2020.

[3] Dr. Robert Klitzman, "Our Next Crisis Will Be Caring for Survivors of Covid-19," *The Washington Post*, June 4, 2020.

[4] Chelsea Janes, Isaac Stanley-Becker, Lenny Bernstein, and Joshua Partlow, "Surge in Virus Hospitalizations Strains Hospitals in Several States," *The Washington Post*, July 8, 2020.

[5] Ibid.

Tamata Kaba

[1] Jennifer Steinhauer, "Frustrated by Lack of Coronavirus Tests, Maryland Got 500,000 From South Korea," *The New York Times*, April 20, 2020.

Shirley Brucelas

[1] Jennifer Steinhauer, Frustrated by Lack of Coronavirus Tests, Maryland Got 500,000 From South Korea. *The New York Times*, April 20, 2020.

[2] Apoorva Mandavilli, "U.S. Plans a Major Shift in Testing Strategy," *The New York Times*, July 2, 2020.

Brenda Halloum

[1] FRONTLINE, "America's Medical Supply Crisis," October 9, 2020.
[2] Ibid.

Patricia Rodriguez

[1] Nicholas Kristof, "Test of Our Lifetimes," WBUR, December 15, 2020.
[2] Ted Amus," Florida's 'Grim Reaper' Lawyer Sued Ron DeSantis over Covid-19. Now the Governor's Attorneys Want Him Sanctioned," *The Washington Post*, December 15, 2020.
[3] Patricia Mazzei, "Whistle Blown, Job Lost, and a Raid on a Scientist," *The New York Times*, December 13, 2020.
[4] Kevin Sieff, "More Americans Are Traveling to Mexico Riviera Maya Than Ever Before. The Parties Have Led to More Coronavirus Cases," *The Washington Post*, December 22, 2020.
[5] "Bleak Commences," *The Economist*, December 12-18, 2020.

Herron Alvarez

[1] Sarah Mervosh, Mike Baker, Patricia Masszei, and Mike Walker, "400,000 Deaths in a Year and Failure at Every Level," *The New York Times*, January 18, 2021.
[2] Simon Romero, "Fighting to Save Lives in Texas, Weary Doctor Counts the Dead," *The New York Times*, February 2, 2021.
[3] David McSwane, "Those of Us Who Don't Die Are Going to Quit; A Crush of Patients, Dwindling Supplies and the Nurse Who Lost Hope," *ProPublica*, December 30, 2020.
[4] Michelle Mahon, "A Deadly Shame, Examining the Physical and Mental Health Impacts of the Pandemic," Zoom Meeting of National Nurses United, at https://www.nationalnursesunited.org/campaign/deadly-shame-report.
[5] "Stars and Gripes," *The Economist*, January 16, 2021.
[6] Denise Brady, Apoorva Mandavilli, and Katie Thomas. "Vaccine Makers Adapt to Battle a Shifting Virus," *The New York Times*, January 26, 2021.

Catherine O'Brien

[1] Sarah Kliff, "Covid Killed His Father. Then Came $1 Million in Medical Expenses," *The New York Times*, May 21, 2021.

[2] Daniela J. Lamas, "Critical Illness's Invisible Scars," *The New York Times*, May 21, 2021.

[3] Sam Sabin, "Exploiting Hospital's Weak Spots," *Politico Future Pulse*, May 21, 2021.

[4] Tatiana Schlossberg, "How Hospital Systems Can Help Their Patients and the Planet," *The New York Times Health Care Media*, May 31, 2021.

[5] Ibid.

[6] Tibisay Zea and Simon Rios, "A 5-Year Boston Area Housing Study Shows How Housing Stability Is Tied to Health Outcomes," WBUR, June 1, 2021.

INDEX

www.ingramcontent.com/pod-product-compliance
Lightning Source LLC
Chambersburg PA
CBHW061011280326

41935CB00009B/925